Emergency Medical Procedures

Designed and edited by
Patient Care Publications, Inc.
Special Publications Group
Patricia B. Hill, Editor

Second edition revised in consultation with:

Elliott L. Cohen, MD, FACEP
Chief, Emergency and Ambulatory Services,
Beverly Hospital, Beverly, Massachusetts

The procedures in this book were developed in consultation with:

David G. Eastman, MD
Emergency Physician, Emergency Out-Patient
Department, Frisbie Memorial Hospital,
Rochester, New Hampshire

G. Gordon Snyder, III, MD, FACS
Associate Professor of Surgery and Lecturer,
Emergency Medical Technician (EMT) Program,
University of Connecticut School of Medicine,
Farmington

Kaye E. Wilkins, MD
Clinical Professor of Orthopedics and Pediatrics,
University of Texas Health Science Center,
San Antonio

Additional review and suggestions were
provided by:

Ad Hoc Committee on Emergency Care Procedures, Emergency Department
Nurses Association

Judith West Pronovost, MN, RN
Department of Nursing in Biological
Dysfunction, University of California
School of Nursing, San Francisco

John C. Bechtler, AEMT-P
Coordinator and Senior Instructor
of Emergency Medical Technicians
State of New York Department of Health

Michael G. Dempsey, D.O.
Specialist in Physical Medicine and Rehabilitation
St. Vincent's Hospital and Medical Center of
New York

EMERGENCY MEDICAL PROCEDURES

for the Home, Auto, & Workplace

Second Revised Edition

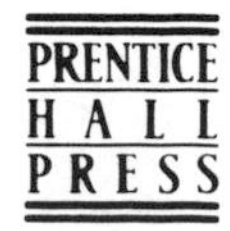
PRENTICE
HALL
PRESS

New York London Toronto Sydney Tokyo Singapore

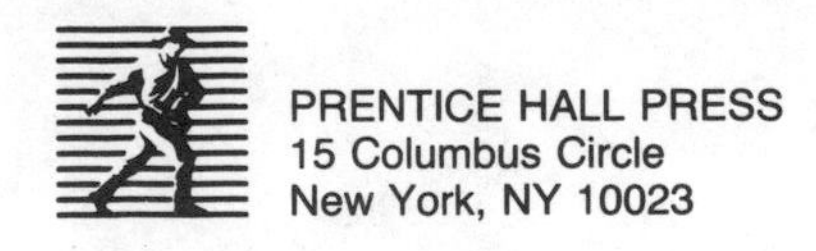

PRENTICE HALL PRESS
15 Columbus Circle
New York, NY 10023

This is a revised edition of a book originally published in 1980 by Prentice-Hall, Inc.

PRENTICE HALL PRESS and colophons are registered trademarks
of Simon & Schuster Inc.

Library of Congress Cataloging-in-Publication Data

Emergency medical procedures for the home, auto, & workplace / Patricia
B. Hill, editor.—2nd rev. ed.
p. cm.—(Emergency medical procedures)
ISBN 0-13-273723-X (pbk.)
1. Medical emergencies—Outlines, syllabi, etc. 2. First aid in
illness and injury—Outlines, syllabi, etc. I. Hill, Patricia B.
II. Series.
RC86.7.E576 1990
616.02'52—dc20 91-22353
CIP

Manufactured in the United States of America

10 9 8 7 6 5 4 3 2 1

The information in this book is not intended to replace instructions by trained professionals. Consult your local emergency-care personnel or physician if at all possible before following the author's proposed courses of emergency treatment. Any application of the treatments set forth in this book is at the reader's discretion and sole risk.

Acknowledgments
The Emergency Medical Procedures series has been developed with the assistance of experts in the fields of first aid, nursing, and medicine. We'd like to thank everyone who was consulted on the various segments of this series, including the consultants listed on page i and:

Lynda R. Applegate, MN, FNP; Gordon A. Benner, MD; Shirley F. Boone, RN, MPH; Timothy Burke, EMT; Richard E. Church, MD; Ruth F. Craven, RN, MN; Lance Feild, MA; George Gomez, EMT, RRT; Deanna Grimes, RN, MPH; Greenwich Health Examiners, Inc.; Alan Kallmann, EMS-I, MS; Patricia D. MacDonald, RN, BSN; Marguerite J. Nick, RN; Cornelia P. Porter, RN, MNEd, PNP; John J. Tobin, MD; John Yost, Fire Chief.

The medical information and procedures in this book represent accepted first aid practices adapted and edited for use in the home or while traveling in a car, truck, van, or recreational vehicle. Consideration has been given to possible delays in obtaining medical assistance. All procedures have been reviewed by the participating consultants as well as other experts in first aid, nursing, and medicine.

Contents

Poisoning

Introduction

These emergency medical procedures have been designed to aid you in managing potentially dangerous or troublesome situations at home, at work, or in your car, truck, van, or recreational vehicle. Whether the problem is an illness, injury, or accident, the Contents will quickly refer you to a specific problem, but it is a good idea for anyone who may be called upon to use the procedures to read through the material before an emergency occurs to get a general idea of the contents and procedures.

Remember that safety and first aid begin with prevention and that the keys to prevention are health maintenance, a well-balanced diet, and moderate, frequent exercise. It is suggested that you or an appropriate authority:

—Periodically review safety principles and rules, paying special attention to the *Basic Emergency Principles and Transfer Procedures* on p. 2. Include children and sitters in these reviews.

—Be on alert for potentially hazardous situations.

—Assemble a first aid kit to be kept with this book, making sure every employee, family member, and sitter knows where it is. The list on p. 1 includes suggested materials for use with these charts.

—Make sure that you and at least one other person in your household take cardiopulmonary resuscitation (CPR) and annual refresher courses. Your local Heart Association or Red Cross chapter can provide information on these courses.

The following recommendations will help you to prevent potential emergencies or to handle those that may occur at home, at work, or on the road despite your precautions.

At Home and Work

—Contact your local fire and/or police department for instructions on emergency evacuation procedures. In areas where hurricanes, tornadoes, and earthquakes are threats, ask where to obtain information on handling such emergencies. All procedures should be adapted to your particular situation and learned by all family members and sitters. Posting these procedures in a central location, along with this book, is also wise.

—Before an emergency occurs, write emergency phone numbers on pages 55–55A of this book. Post copies of these numbers by every phone. Teach young children the emergency or ambulance number and the fire or police number and how to dial them.

On the Road

—Practice good driving habits: Don't drive when tired or under the influence of alcohol or drugs, and don't rely on caffeine or other stimulants to keep you awake. Stay alert and drive defensively.

—Keep your vehicle in good working condition.

—Limit driving when road conditions are hazardous.

—Make it a rule, particularly when road conditions are hazardous, to note the last emergency call box, home, or open business.

—Assemble a vehicular emergency kit that includes warning lights or flares, a flashlight, emergency signs, and glass cleaner.

—Consider investing in a CB radio if you do not already own one.

—If you live in or are traveling to an area with potentially dangerous climatic or geographical factors, learn and teach others traveling with you how to deal with problems that may arise. For example, in cold weather when confined to a vehicle because of a flat tire, accident, snow, or other reason, use blankets and body heat for warmth; keep the exhaust pipe clear of snow, dirt, and other matter; and run the engine and heater for only

10 minutes every hour. Running the engine more frequently may result in asphyxiation.
—Before an emergency occurs, read *Arrival at the Scene of an Accident* on p. 3.

When a medical emergency occurs:

Remain calm. Take a deep breath, then read these instructions. With all emergencies, except when there is no pulse (then turn immediately to *CPR,* pp. 5–7), one or two minutes spent getting the situation under control will improve your effectiveness.
Look up the major problem in the Contents. If a serious emergency occurs that you cannot find listed, the best procedure is to obtain emergency or medical assistance.
Provide only emergency care outlined in these charts unless you receive instructions for additional care from a medically trained person via telephone, radio, or other means.
Use common sense with these charts; only you know your particular situation. The primary rule of emergency aid is to cause no further injury. Most important during any medical emergency—Remember your ABCs:
—Make sure the *airway* is unobstructed.
—Make sure the person is *breathing.*
—Be sure the *circulation* of blood is maintained.
(Heart is kept pumping, bleeding is controlled, etc.)

Getting Help

When you are faced with an emergency situation, you will have to use your own judgment about how to get help. When emergency assistance is necessary, you will have to decide, particularly in a vehicular emergency, whether it is best to summon help or drive the person to an emergency room. When a person is sick or injured while riding in a vehicle, you will have to decide also whether the person can be cared for without stopping or whether care can best be given by pulling off the road or to a nearby home or business. When you need additional assistance, whether at home or on the road, uso one or more of the following:
—*Telephone:* A telephone is your best means of getting help. On the road, don't forget such sources of telephones as an emergency call box, a home, or an open business.
—*Radio:* Use any two-way radio, such as a CB. On a CB, emergencies are reported on channel 9. On the road, if you don't have a radio, flag down a taxi, delivery truck, or private motorist with a CB or car phone.

In addition to the above, the following distress signals may be used and are particularly geared to emergencies which may occur while driving in sparsely populated areas:
—*Standard Ground-to-Air Signals:* As large as possible, illustrate by digging in dirt or snow or use tree limbs, rocks, clothing, etc. Be sure the symbols contrast the ground color as much as possible.

▌ for "Require doctor—serious injuries"

▌▌ for "Require medical supplies"

—*Universal Distress Signals:* A series of three sights or sounds, such as shouts, blows on a whistle or horn, high-frequency beeps, gunshots, or flashes of light.
—*SOS Morse Code Distress Signal:* A series of three dots, three dashes, three dots made by blows on a whistle or horn, high-frequency beeps, or flashes of light.

· · · — — — · · · means SOS or Help!

—*A large flag* at the top of a tree or hung on an antenna— the brighter, the better.
—*A mirror or other shiny object* flashed across the sky several times a day to attract planes.
—*Flares*

1 Basic Medical Supplies

Basic Medical Supplies for Use with the Emergency Medical Procedures

The supplies specified are divided into two lists: one consists of medical supplies, which should be kept separate for emergency care and first aid; the other consists of cooking or basic supplies, which may be used for other purposes as well as for emergencies. The designated provisions include only those supplies required in these charts. Most of these items are available in supermarkets or pharmacies.

The two lists should meet the needs for treating injuries or illnesses most frequently encountered in the home, at work, or on the road. However, if anyone in your household, workplace, or vehicle has a history of allergic reaction to insect stings, or if you live, work, or are traveling in an area densely inhabited by insects, we recommend that you include an insect-bite kit, available by prescription from your physician. It is also advisable to include a snakebite kit in regions populated by poisonous snakes.

Many of the suggested materials are marked with an (*) to indicate that they are not crucial and/or feasible for a *vehicle* medical supply kit. Unless you will be driving in an area that is very isolated, it is assumed that these supplies would be readily obtainable at at nearby home, store, or other business.

Medical Supplies
activated charcoal powder (medicinal)
adhesive tape (1 inch)
antacids (Gelusil, Maalox, Mylanta)*
antihistamine (Benadryl)
aspirin and acetaminophen (Tylenol, Datril)
Betadine solution
calamine lotion*
cold pack
cotton swabs*
elastic bandage (3 inch)
Epsom salts*
fever thermometer*
insect-bite kit**
lip balm (ChapStick, etc.)*
oil of cloves*
petroleum jelly (Vaseline, etc.)*
pocket mask (for CPR)
razor blade*
rubbing alcohol
scissors
smelling salts (ammonia capsules)*
snakebite kit***
sterile gauze bandage (3 inch)
sterile gauze pads (4 × 4 inches)
syrup of ipecac
thermal blanket
topical antibiotic ointment (Triple-Antibiotic Ointment, Neosporin, Bacitracin, etc.)
tweezers
vaporizer (preferably cold-steam)*

Cooking and Basic Supplies that can be used as Medical Supplies
aluminum foil
baking soda
blankets
bouillon cubes
candle or paraffin*
clean cloth (pieces of sheeting)
cup
drinking water*
flashlight
fruit juices (with sugar added)*
honey*
meat tenderizer*
milk*
plastic bags
plastic wrap
salt
soap (without deodorant, cold cream)*
soft drinks (sugar-sweetened)*
sugar (loose)*
tea*
towels*
wire cutters*

*Not crucial and/or feasible for a *vehicle* medical supply kit unless in a very isolated area.
**If someone is allergic to stings.
***If in an area inhabited by poisonous snakes.

2 Basic Emergency Principles & Transfer Procedures

Use these principles and procedures only if trained emergency personnel are not available.

1. If necessary:
   —Clear mouth of foreign matter and establish open airway.
   —Check breathing and carotid (neck) pulse. If no breathing or pulse, see *Artificial Respiration/ CPR,* pp. 4–7.
   —Control bleeding. (See p. 50.)
2. **Do not** move sick or injured person, particularly with back or neck injury, unless:
   —location is dangerous (i.e., fire, threat of explosion, etc.) or
   —crucial emergency care cannot be given at present location.
3. If person is unconscious from direct blow to head or a fall, assume neck, and possibly back, injury. (See p. 29.)
4. —Check for injuries and immobilize all injured parts, if possible.
   —**Do not** straighten fractured or dislocated limbs unless circulation is impaired and emergency aid will not be available within 15 minutes.
   —**Do not** remove objects imbedded deeply in person (i.e., knife, pencil) and **do not** remove person who is stuck on an object (i.e. fence post, stick shift). Instead, immobilize person and object to prevent further injury. If moving is necessary, disassemble or shorten object and transport person with imbedded object immobilized.
   —Avoid jarring person unnecessarily while preparing for transfer.
   —Always transport injured person lying down; person with shortness of breath may be more comfortable in sitting position.
5. Obtain assistance whenever possible before moving sick or injured person.

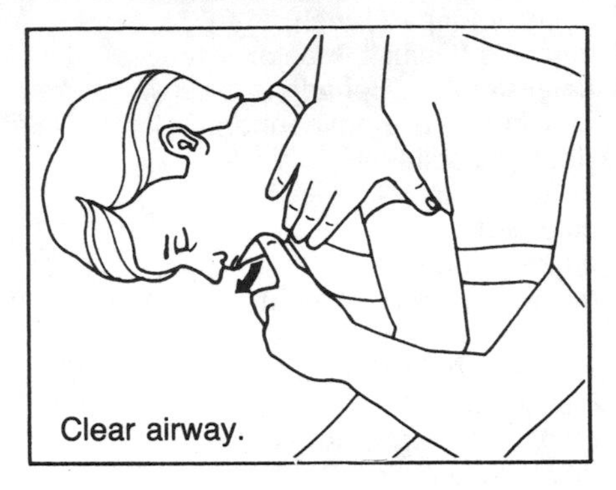
Clear airway.

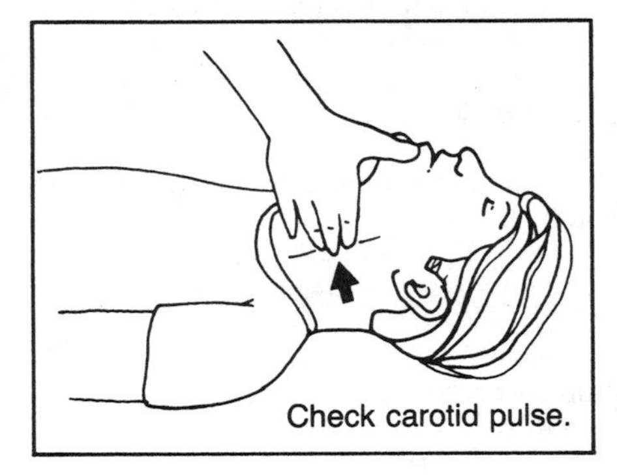
Check carotid pulse.

If possibility of back and/or neck injury, see p. 29.

How many rescuers are there?

One

Two or more (see next page).

Is the person injured, having a heart attack, or unconscious?

No → Place person's arm around your neck and support person at waist. Slowly assist to safety. If person is too heavy or too weak, use blanket or clothes drag. (See A or B below.)

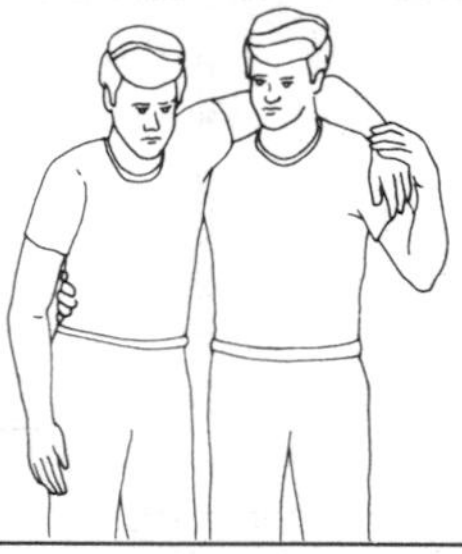

Yes ↓

Is a stretcher, board, or blanket available?

No → B

Yes → A

A

—Lay it along the person's most in-ured side. (If using blanket, gather it in lengthwise folds.)
—Grasp person at hips and shoulders, and gently roll onto least injured side.
—Slide board or blanket underneath.
—Roll person onto other side, pulling blanket under, then roll onto back.
—Grasp board or blanket under person's head and neck and pull person vertically to safety, keeping blanket low to ground.

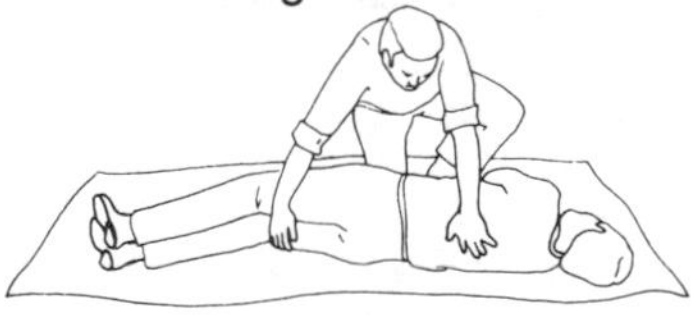

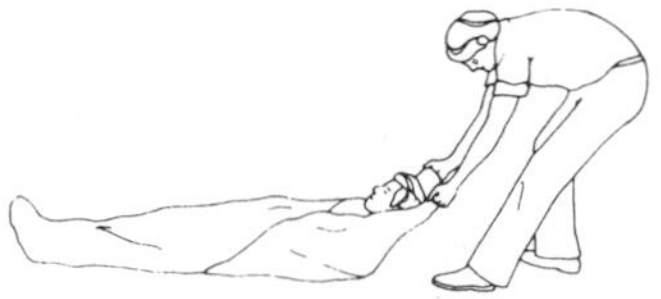

B

Place person on back. Stand at person's head, supporting head at back of neck. Slowly drag person to safety, keeping person low to ground. **Do not** pull clothing so tight that it blocks airway.

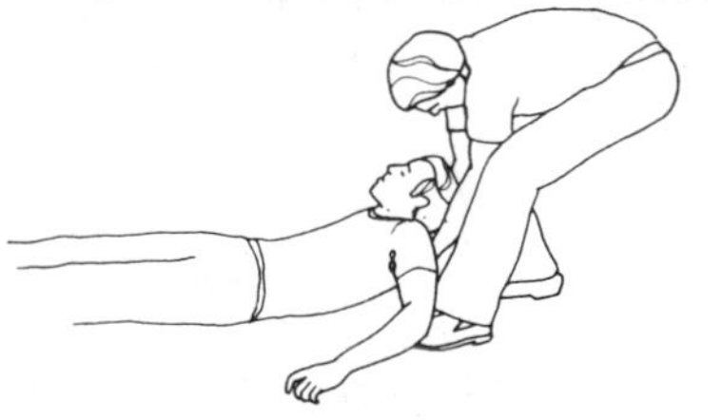

Remain calm; assess the situation. See *Contents* for appropriate chart. Speak quietly to reassure sick or injured person.

2A Transfer Procedures (cont.)

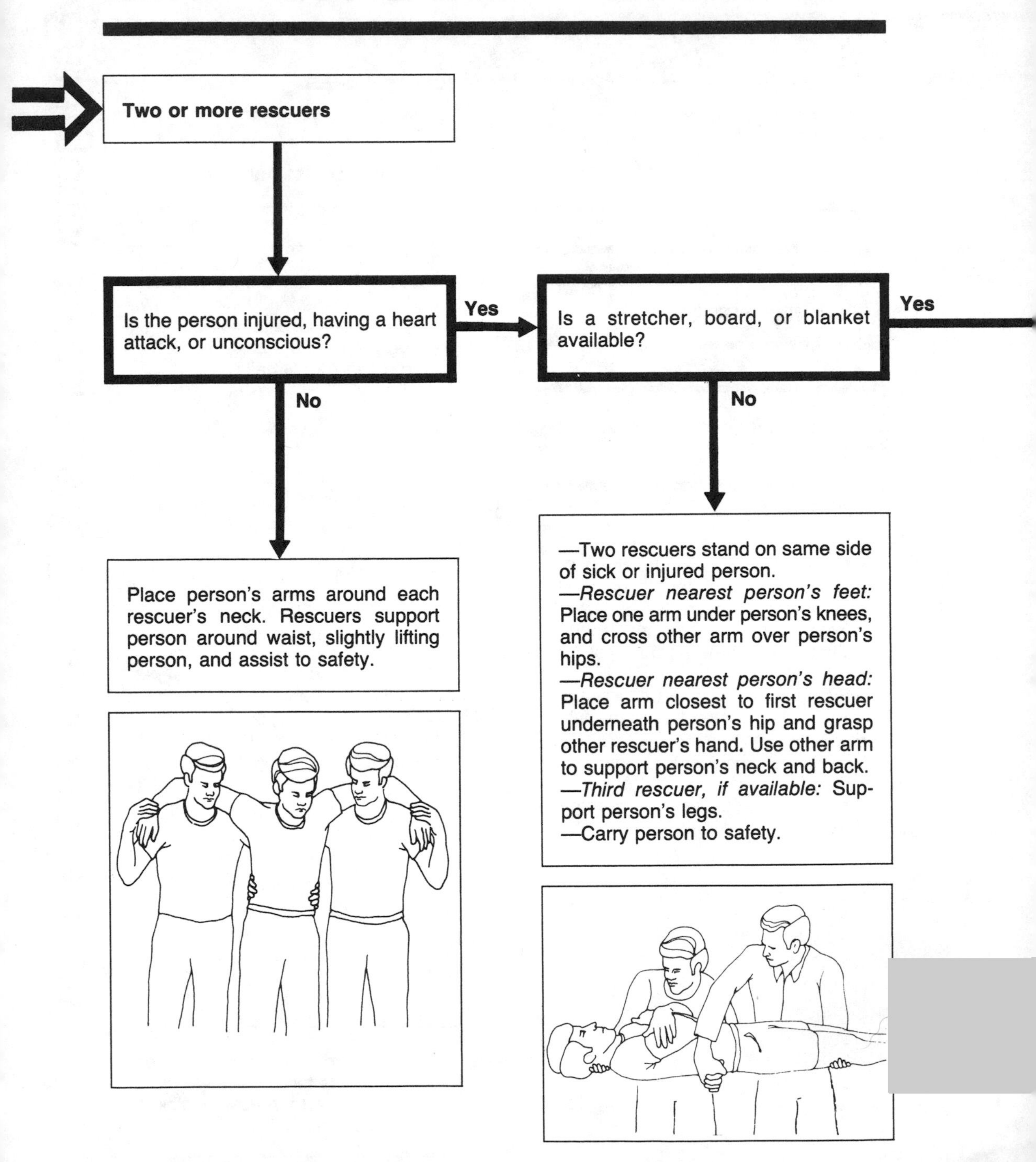

Two or more rescuers
Is the person injured, having a heart attack, or unconscious?
Yes
No
Is a stretcher, board, or blanket available?
Yes
No
Place person's arms around each rescuer's neck. Rescuers support person around waist, slightly lifting person, and assist to safety.
—Two rescuers stand on same side of sick or injured person.
—*Rescuer nearest person's feet:* Place one arm under person's knees, and cross other arm over person's hips.
—*Rescuer nearest person's head:* Place arm closest to first rescuer underneath person's hip and grasp other rescuer's hand. Use other arm to support person's neck and back.
—*Third rescuer, if available:* Support person's legs.
—Carry person to safety.

—Lay it along the person's most injured side. (If using blanket, gather it in lengthwise folds.)
—Grasp person at hips and shoulders, and gently roll onto least injured side.
—Slide board underneath, then gently roll person on back.
—Rescuers stand on either side of person, lift slowly and simultaneously, and carry to safety.

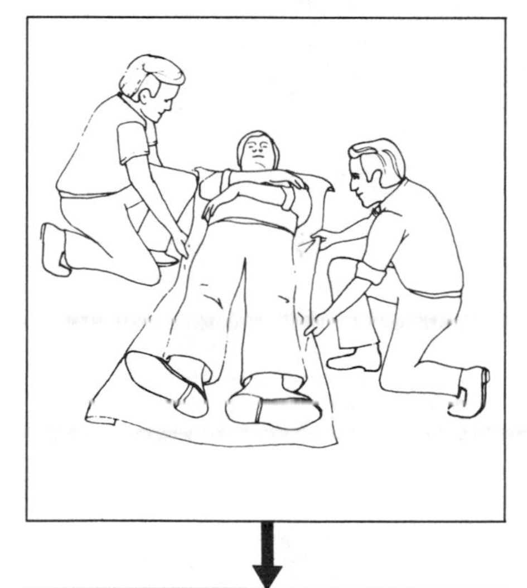

Remain calm; assess the situation. See *Contents* for appropriate chart. Speak quietly to reassure sick or injured person.

3 Arrival at the Scene of an Accident
(When assistance has not already arrived)

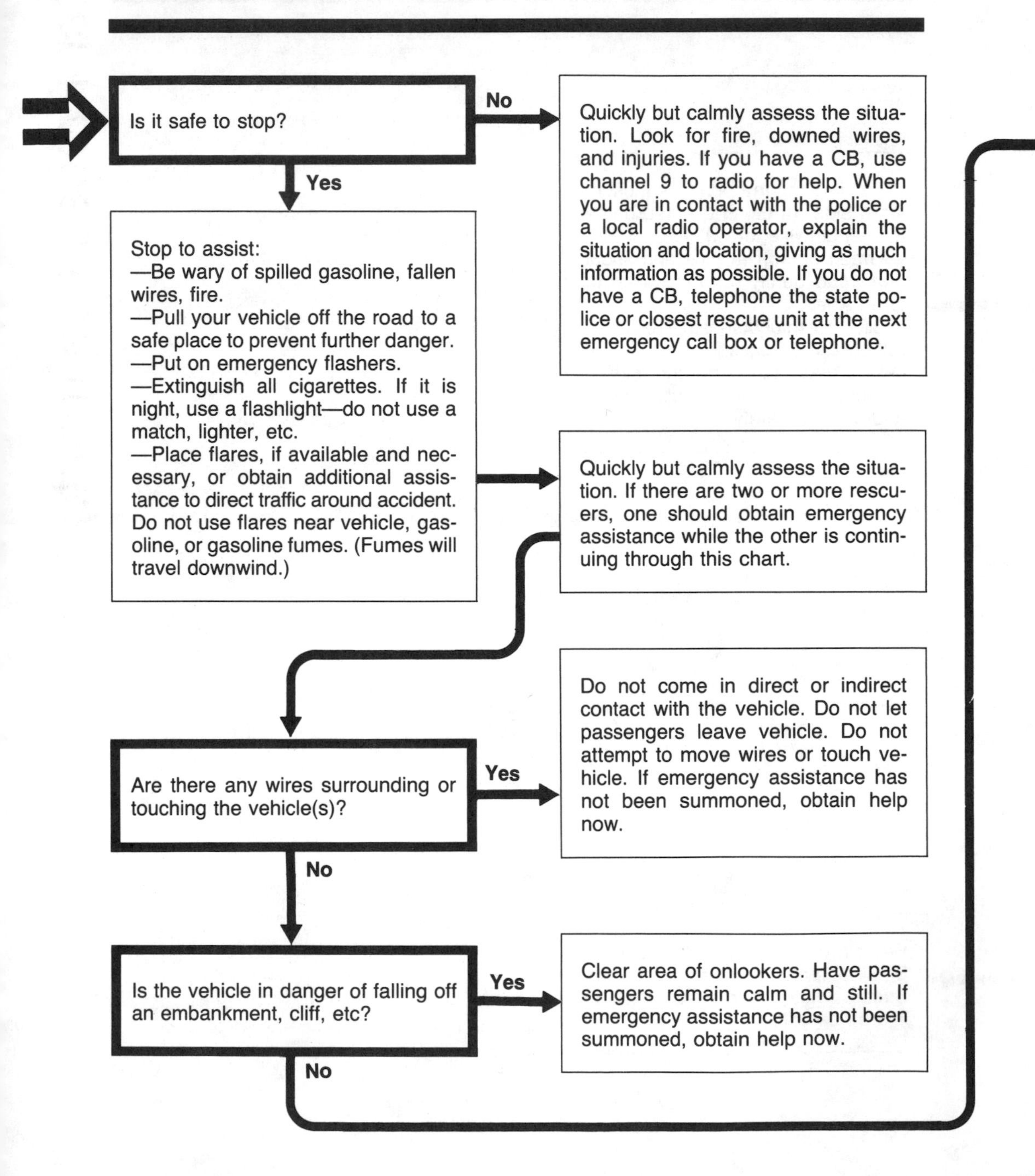

Is it safe to stop?
No
Quickly but calmly assess the situation. Look for fire, downed wires, and injuries. If you have a CB, use channel 9 to radio for help. When you are in contact with the police or a local radio operator, explain the situation and location, giving as much information as possible. If you do not have a CB, telephone the state police or closest rescue unit at the next emergency call box or telephone.
Yes
Stop to assist:
—Be wary of spilled gasoline, fallen wires, fire.
—Pull your vehicle off the road to a safe place to prevent further danger.
—Put on emergency flashers.
—Extinguish all cigarettes. If it is night, use a flashlight—do not use a match, lighter, etc.
—Place flares, if available and necessary, or obtain additional assistance to direct traffic around accident. Do not use flares near vehicle, gasoline, or gasoline fumes. (Fumes will travel downwind.)
Quickly but calmly assess the situation. If there are two or more rescuers, one should obtain emergency assistance while the other is continuing through this chart.
Are there any wires surrounding or touching the vehicle(s)?
Yes
Do not come in direct or indirect contact with the vehicle. Do not let passengers leave vehicle. Do not attempt to move wires or touch vehicle. If emergency assistance has not been summoned, obtain help now.
No
Is the vehicle in danger of falling off an embankment, cliff, etc?
Yes
Clear area of onlookers. Have passengers remain calm and still. If emergency assistance has not been summoned, obtain help now.
No

Never right an overturned vehicle or do anything else which may cause further injury or danger unless directed to do so below or by trained emergency or medical authorities.

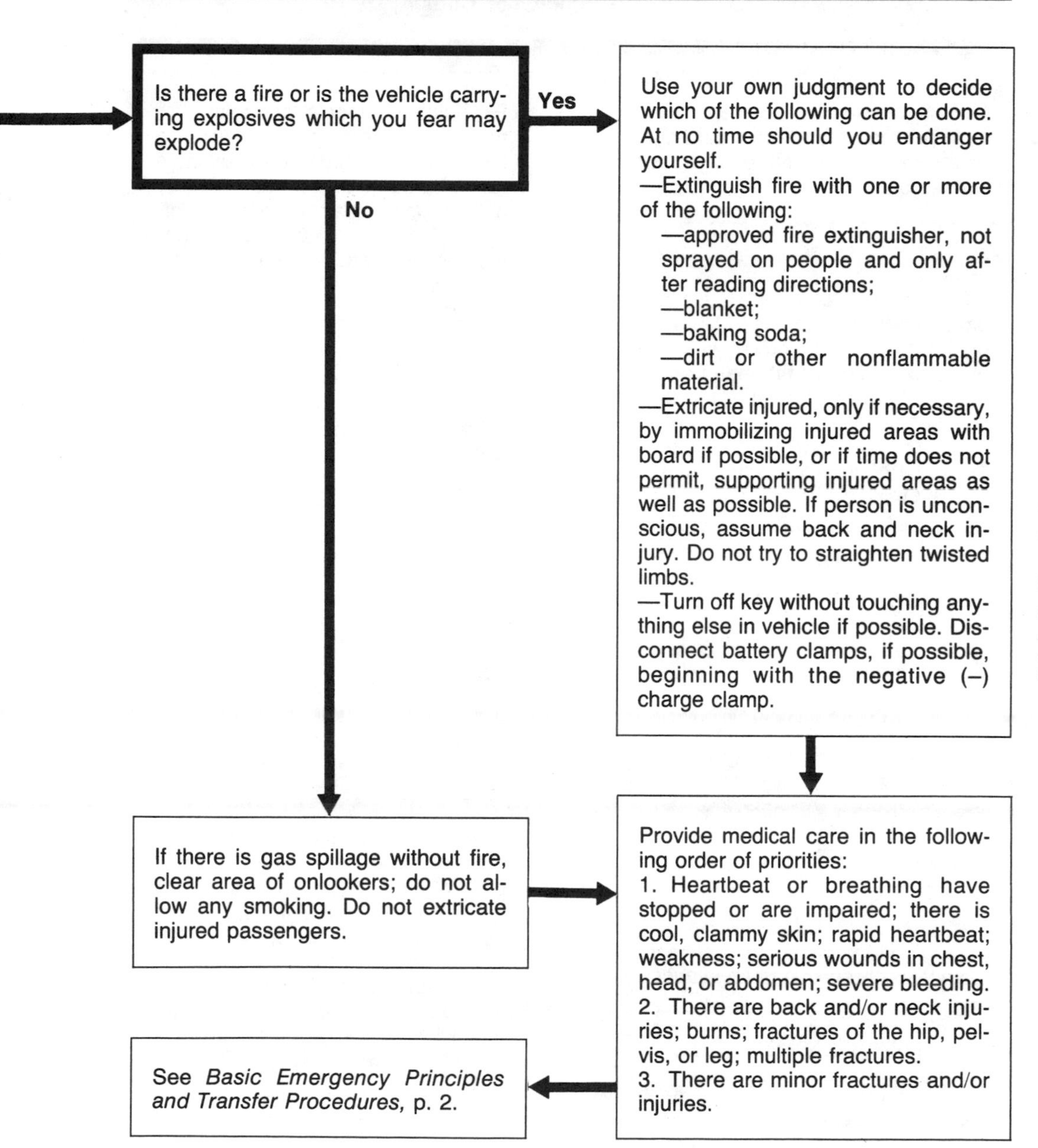
Is there a fire or is the vehicle carrying explosives which you fear may explode?
Yes
No
Use your own judgment to decide which of the following can be done. At no time should you endanger yourself.
—Extinguish fire with one or more of the following:
—approved fire extinguisher, not sprayed on people and only after reading directions;
—blanket;
—baking soda;
—dirt or other nonflammable material.
—Extricate injured, only if necessary, by immobilizing injured areas with board if possible, or if time does not permit, supporting injured areas as well as possible. If person is unconscious, assume back and neck injury. Do not try to straighten twisted limbs.
—Turn off key without touching anything else in vehicle if possible. Disconnect battery clamps, if possible, beginning with the negative (–) charge clamp.
If there is gas spillage without fire, clear area of onlookers; do not allow any smoking. Do not extricate injured passengers.
Provide medical care in the following order of priorities:
1. Heartbeat or breathing have stopped or are impaired; there is cool, clammy skin; rapid heartbeat; weakness; serious wounds in chest, head, or abdomen; severe bleeding.
2. There are back and/or neck injuries; burns; fractures of the hip, pelvis, or leg; multiple fractures.
3. There are minor fractures and/or injuries.
See Basic Emergency Principles and Transfer Procedures, p. 2.

4 Artificial Respiration (Rescue Breathing)

This chart should only be used if the person is not breathing, but his heart is beating. Check the neck carefully for a carotid pulse; it may be very faint. If the person has no pulse, see *CPR*, pp. 5–7. Artificial respiration and CPR should be performed even if a person has been under water for up to 60 minutes. If the person choked before breathing stopped, see *Choking*, p. 10.

Make sure person is not responsive. Turn person on back on a hard surface. Be careful not to cause or worsen a neck injury.

For an adult or older child, use one hand to gently lift person's chin while pushing forehead down with the other hand. **Do not tilt head back if neck is injured.*** *For an infant,* support upper back with hand or folded sheet or towel and gently lift chin forward, **unless neck is injured. Do not overextend neck.**

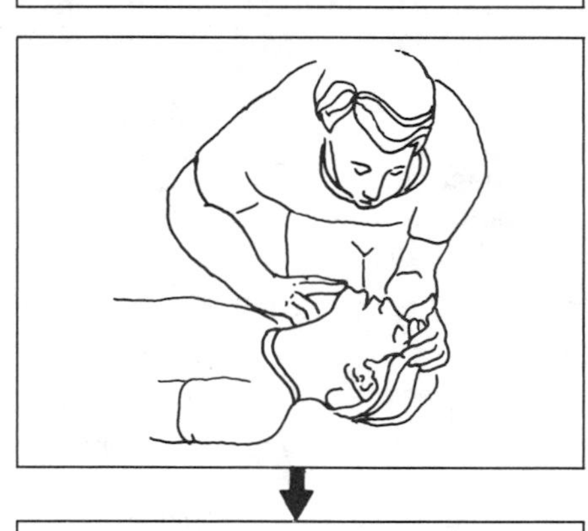

For an adult pinch nostrils with fingers of hand resting on forehead. Do not pinch nostrils of an *infant*.

Continue to lift chin, take a deep breath, and seal your mouth tightly around person's mouth or over nose and mouth in infants (or use pocket mask if available).

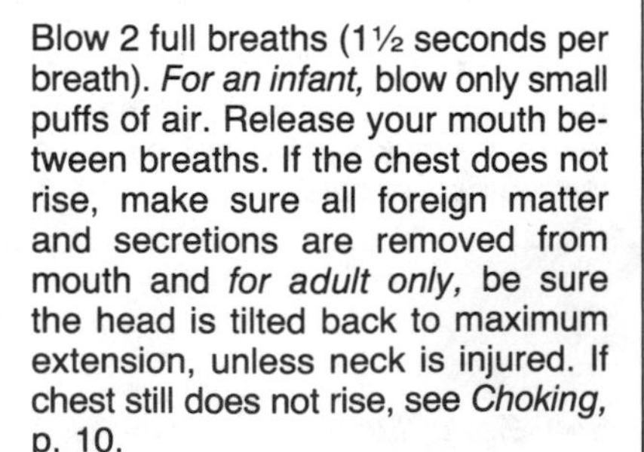

Blow 2 full breaths (1½ seconds per breath). *For an infant,* blow only small puffs of air. Release your mouth between breaths. If the chest does not rise, make sure all foreign matter and secretions are removed from mouth and *for adult only,* be sure the head is tilted back to maximum extension, unless neck is injured. If chest still does not rise, see *Choking,* p. 10.

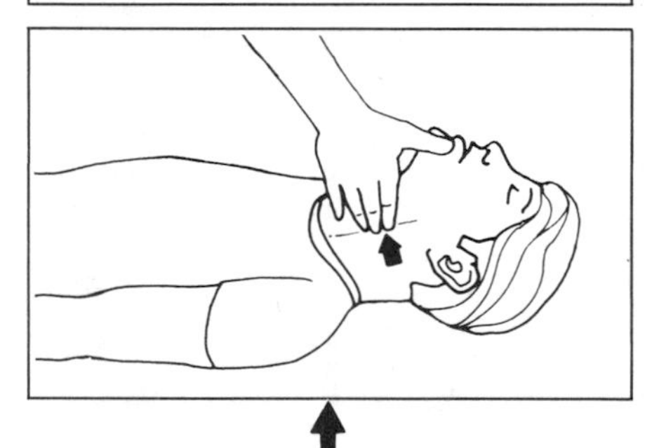

Feel neck for 5–10 seconds for a carotid pulse. If there is none, see *CPR,* pp. 5–7.

Reposition person's head and repeat 2 breaths. Continue ventilation for *adults* and *older children* at a rate of 1 every 5 seconds—1 every 3 seconds for infants, checking carotid pulse every 1–2 minutes, until the person breathes regularly without assistance.

If gas or smoke is present, move person to safety.

The first thing you must do if the person appears unconscious is to determine unresponsiveness by shaking the person while asking, "Are you okay?" If the person does not respond, shout for help even if you think you are alone. If there are two or more rescuers, one should obtain emergency assistance while the other is following the procedures outlined below.

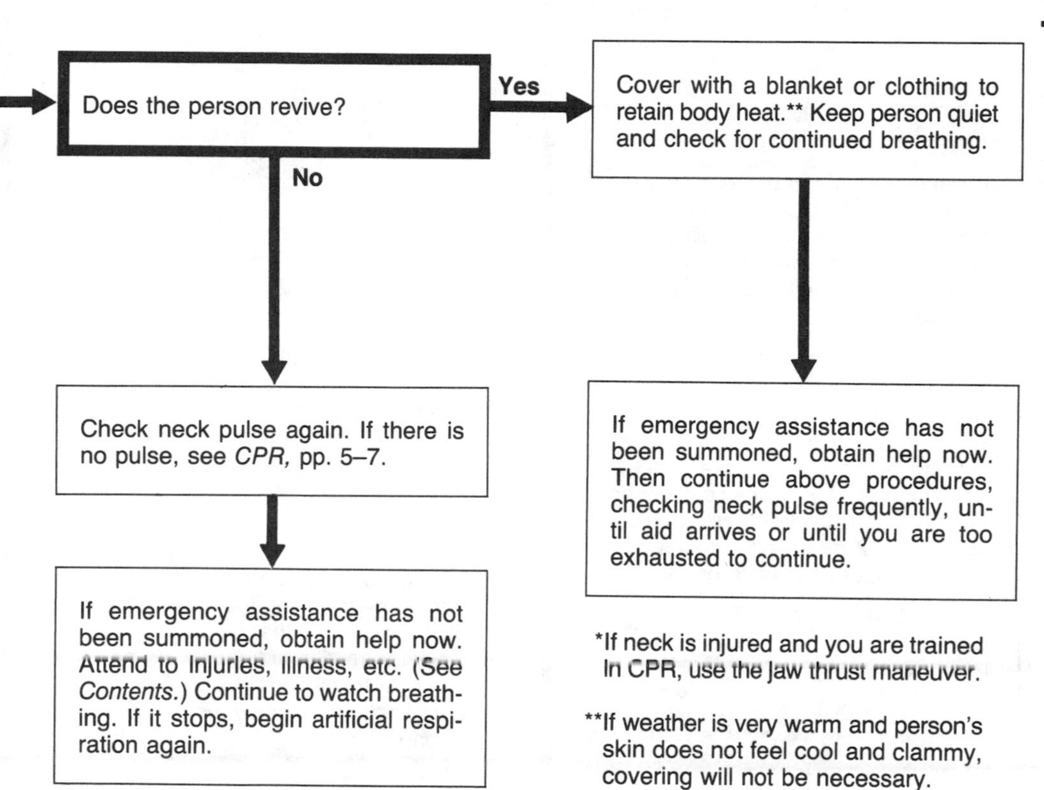
Does the person revive?
Yes
Cover with a blanket or clothing to retain body heat.** Keep person quiet and check for continued breathing.
No
Check neck pulse again. If there is no pulse, see CPR, pp. 5–7.
If emergency assistance has not been summoned, obtain help now. Then continue above procedures, checking neck pulse frequently, until aid arrives or until you are too exhausted to continue.
If emergency assistance has not been summoned, obtain help now. Attend to injuries, illness, etc. (See Contents.) Continue to watch breathing. If it stops, begin artificial respiration again.

*If neck is injured and you are trained in CPR, use the jaw thrust maneuver.

**If weather is very warm and person's skin does not feel cool and clammy, covering will not be necessary.

CPR
(1 Rescuer)

For infants, see *CPR (Infants)*, p. 7.

If 2 or more rescuers, see p. 6. **Begin CPR immediately. Do not use CPR on a person who has a pulse. It may cause serious complications. Check the neck artery carefully; pulse may be weak. If there is a pulse but no sign of breathing, see *Artificial Respiration*, p. 4.**

Place person flat on back on floor or ground. Ask "Are you all right?" two or three times. If person is not aroused, lightly shake or slap. Shout for help, even if you think you are alone.

Kneel at side of head. Open airway. Remove any foreign materials from mouth and gently lift chin while pushing forehead down with other hand. **Do not push head back if neck is injured.***

Pinch nostrils together and rest palm of hand on forehead. Take a deep breath and seal your lips tightly over mouth, or use pocket mask if available. Blow 2 deep, full breaths, releasing mouth after each breath.

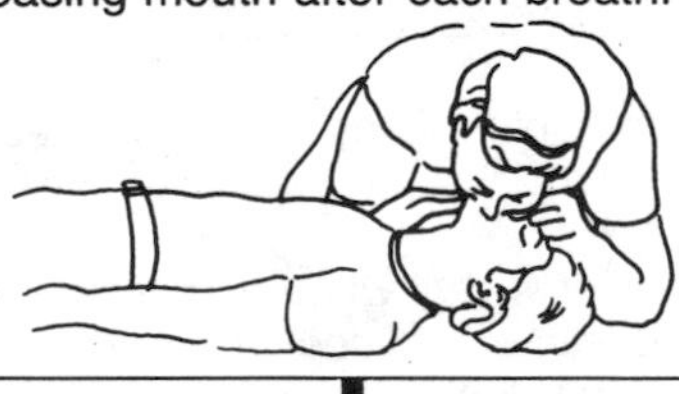

Feel for pulse for 5–10 seconds. Check the neck artery carefully; pulse may be weak. If there is a pulse, but breathing is weak or absent, continue only ventilation at a rate of 1 every 5 seconds until person revives.

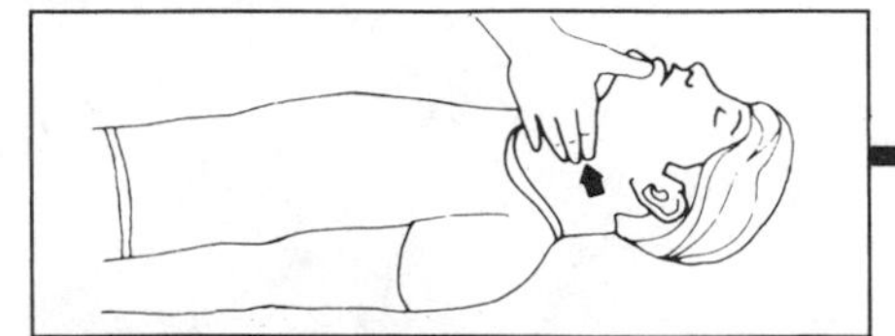

If no pulse, follow rib cage up to center of chest. Place index and middle finger on tip of breastbone.

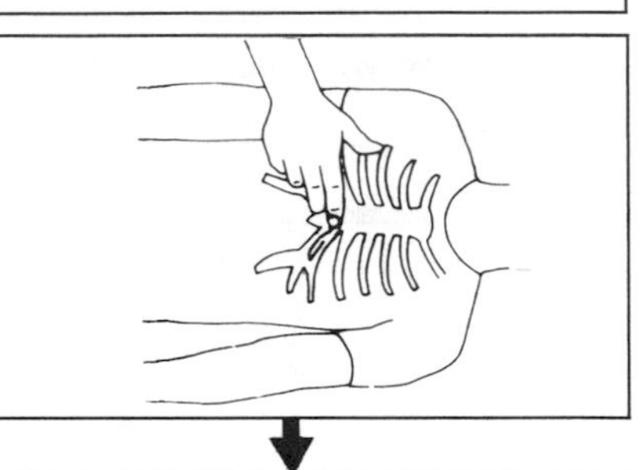

Place heel of other hand immediately next to and touching the index finger. Make sure it is directly centered over the breastbone.

For adults, and children over 80 pounds only, place heel of the first hand directly over the wrist of the other hand on the person's lower breastbone. Clasp fingers and bend those of lower hand back. *For children under 80 pounds,* use only heel of one hand.

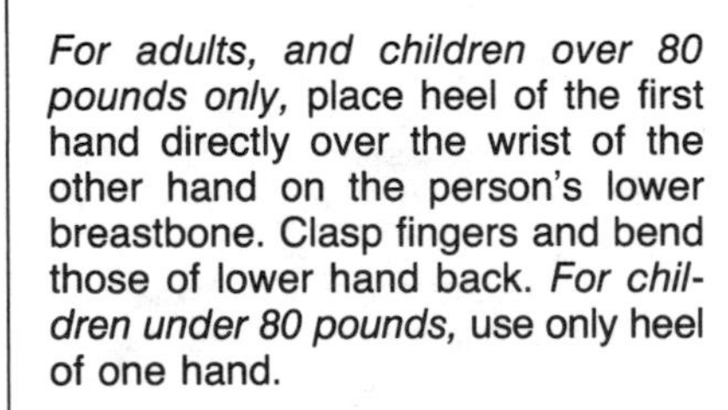

Lean directly over the person and straighten your arm(s).

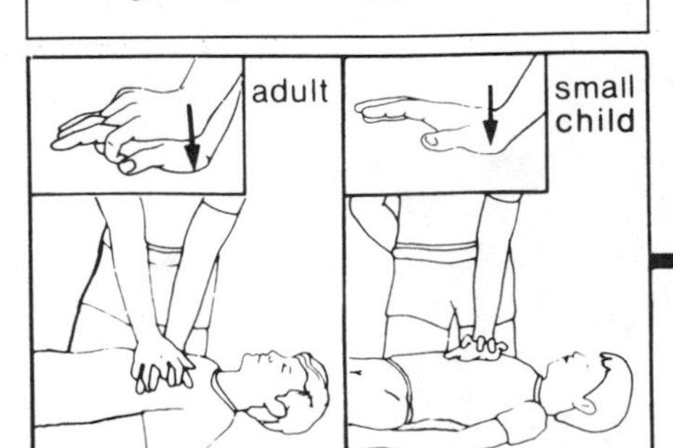
adult
small child

Although the necessary fundamentals for performing CPR are set forth on this chart, there is no substitute for a course in CPR given by a certified instructor.

Use straight-down pressure through both arms (one arm for child under 80 pounds) to push breastbone against heart. *For an adult,* depress breastbone 1½″ to 2″; *for a child,* ¾″ to 1½″.

↓

The compression/relaxation combination is performed at a rate of 80–100 times per minute. Count one-and-two-and-three, etc. Completely release pressure during relaxation phase without lifting your hand(s) from person's chest.

↓

After 15 compressions, breathe twice into the mouth. Repeat the 15-to-2 cycle 4 times.

↓

Are breathing and pulse restored?

No →

Check breathing and neck pulse carefully. If no pulse, continue CPR. Check for pulse and breathing every 4–6 cycles until the person is revived, help arrives, or you can no longor oontinuo. If thoro io a puloo, but breathing is weak or absent, continue only ventilation at a rate of 1 every 5 seconds until person revives. Continue to monitor pulse closely.

↓

Yes ↓

Loosen clothing to relieve pressure. Keep person warm and check for continued breathing and pulse.

→

If emergency assistance has not been summoned, obtain help now. Attend to injuries, illness, etc. (See *Contents.*)

*If neck is injured and you are trained in CPR, use jaw thrust maneuver.

CPR

(2 or More Rescuers)

For infants, see CPR (*Infants*), p. 7.

If only one rescuer, see p. 5. Rescuers read chart before beginning CPR. If 3 or more rescuers, 2 begin CPR while the other obtains emergency assistance. Rescuers kneel at opposite sides of person, one at chest, one at head.

Place person flat on back on floor or ground. Ask "Are you all right?" two or three times. If person is not aroused, lightly shake or slap.

Open airway. Remove any foreign materials from mouth. Gently lift chin while pushing forehead down with other hand. **Do not tilt head back if neck is injured and do not overextend neck.***

Rescuer 1: Pinch nostrils together and rest palm of hand on forehead. Take a deep breath and seal your lips tightly over mouth, or use pocket mask if available. Blow 2 deep, full breaths, releasing mouth after each breath.

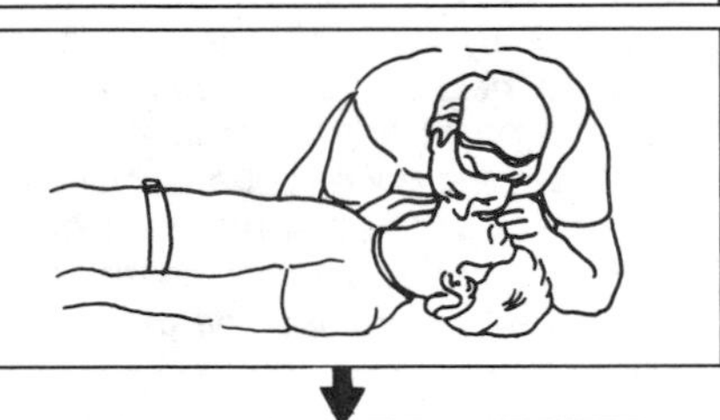

Feel for pulse for 5–10 seconds. Check the neck artery carefully; pulse may be weak. If there is a pulse, but breathing is weak or absent, continue only ventilation at a rate of 1 every 5 seconds until person revives.

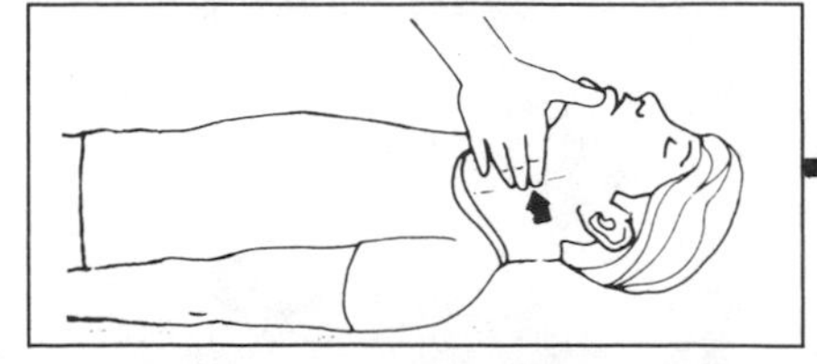

If no pulse, **Rescuer 2:** Follow rib cage up to center of chest. Place index and middle finger on tip of breastbone.

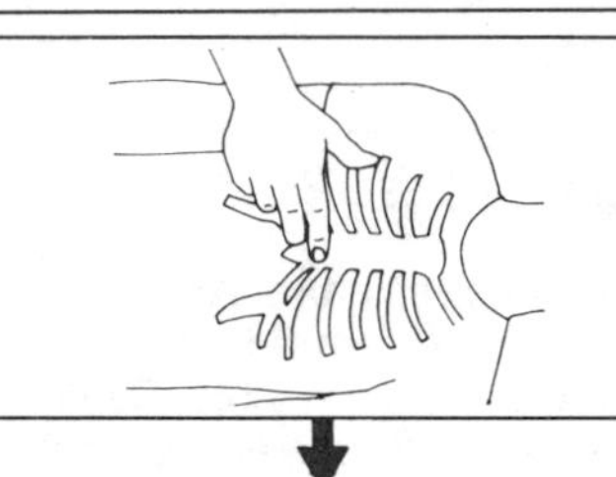

Place heel of other hand immediately next to and touching the index finger. Make sure it is directly centered over the breastbone.

For adults and children over 80 pounds only, place heel of the first hand directly over the wrist of the other hand on the person's lower breastbone. Clasp fingers and bend those of lower hand back. *For children under 80 pounds,* use only heel of one hand.

Lean directly over the person and straighten your arm(s).

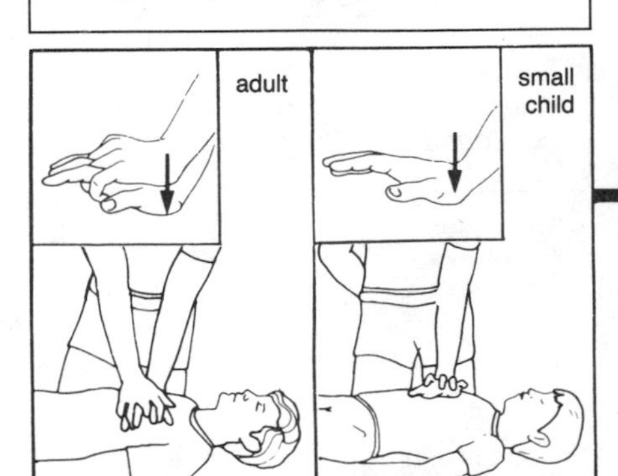
adult
small child

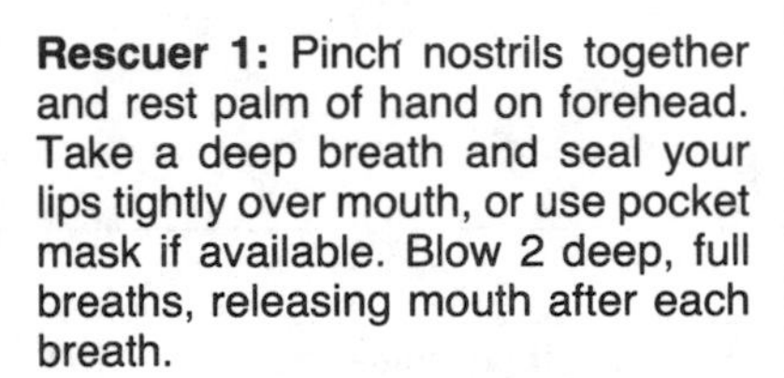

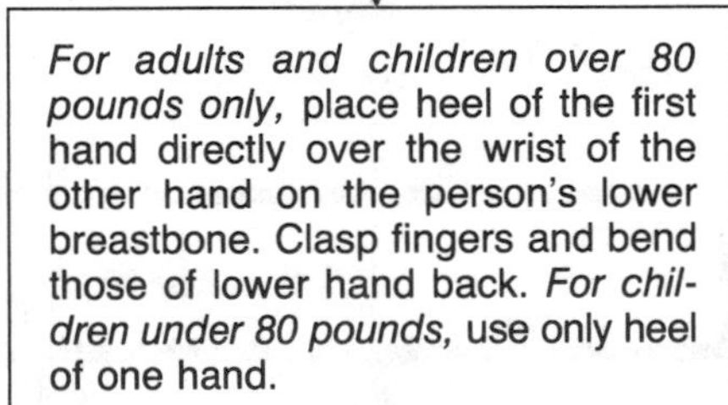

Begin CPR immediately. Do not use CPR on a person who has a pulse. It may cause serious complications. Check neck artery carefully; pulse may be weak. If there is a pulse but no sign of breathing, see *Artificial Respiration*, p. 4.

Although the necessary fundamentals for performing CPR are set forth on this chart, there is no substitute for a course in CPR given by a certified instructor.

→ Use straight-down pressure through both arms (one arm for child under 80 pounds) to push breastbone against heart. *For an adult,* depress breastbone 1½″ to 2″; *for a child,* ¾″ to 1½″.

↓

The compression/relaxation combination is performed at a rate of 80–100 per minute. Count one-and-two-and-three-and, etc., out loud. Completely release pressure during the relaxation phase, without lifting your hand(s) from person's chest.

↓

After the fourth compression, **Rescuer 1** takes a deep breath. After the fifth compression, he seals his mouth tightly over person's mouth, pinches the nostrils, and blows once. Repeat the 5-to-1 cycle for about a minute.

↓

Does the person revive?

No → Check breathing and neck pulse carefully. If no pulse, continue CPR. Change positions when compressor becomes tired. Check for pulse and breathing every few minutes until person is revived, help arrives, or you can no longer continue.

↓

If there is a pulse, but breathing is weak or absent, continue only ventilation at a rate of 1 every 5 seconds until person revives. Continue to monitor pulse closely.

↓

If emergency assistance has not been summoned, obtain help now. Attend to injuries, illness, etc. (See *Contents*.)

Yes → Loosen clothing to relieve pressure. Keep person warm and check for continued breathing and pulse. → If emergency assistance has not been summoned, obtain help now.

*If neck is injured and you are trained in CPR, use the jaw thrust maneuver.

7 CPR
(Infants)

Begin CPR immediately. If 2 or more rescuers, 1 begin CPR while other gets help. Do not use CPR on an infant whose heart is beating. It may cause serious complications. Check carefully above left nipple for heartbeat; pulse may be weak. If there is a heartbeat but no sign of breathing, see *Artificial Respiration*, p. 4.

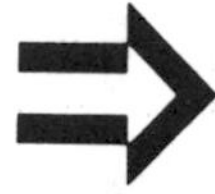

Place infant flat on back. Call child's name two or three times; try to arouse by lightly shaking or tapping hard on bottom of bare foot. Shout for help even if you think you are alone.

Open airway. Remove any foreign materials from mouth. Gently lift chin slightly, supporting upper back with hand or folded sheet or towel. **Do not tilt head back if neck is injured and do not overextend neck.***

Seal your mouth over infant's mouth and nose and blow 2 puffs of air.

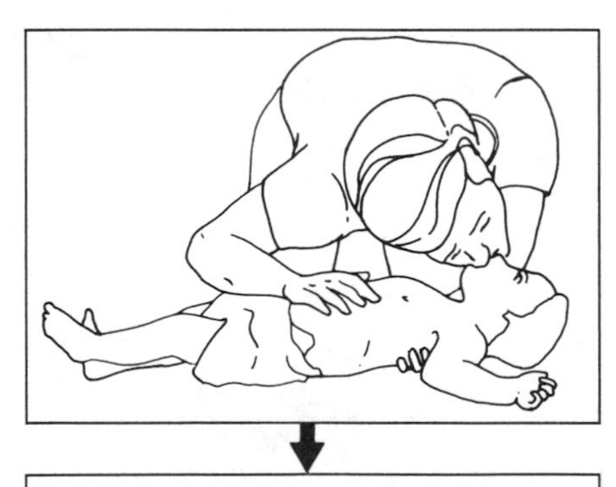

Feel for pulse above left nipple for 5–10 seconds. Check carefully; pulse may be weak. If there is a pulse, but breathing is weak or absent, continue only ventilation at a rate of 1 every 3 seconds until infant revives.

If no pulse, spread one hand over chest so that thumb is at base of throat and little finger is at end of breastbone. Keep index finger and middle finger together and lift others from chest.

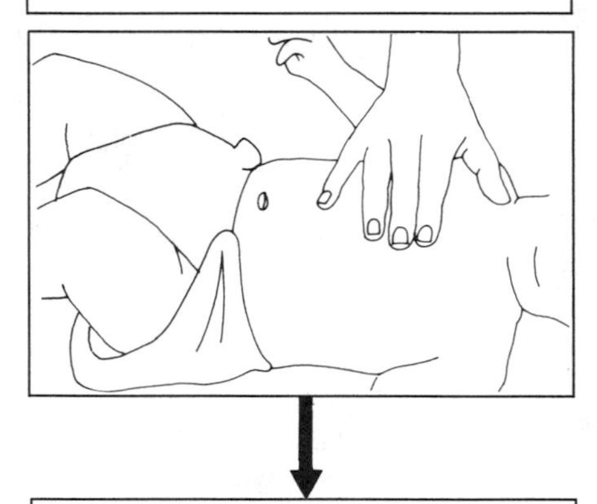

With tips of index finger and middle finger press gently on center of breastbone, depressing ½″ to ¾″.

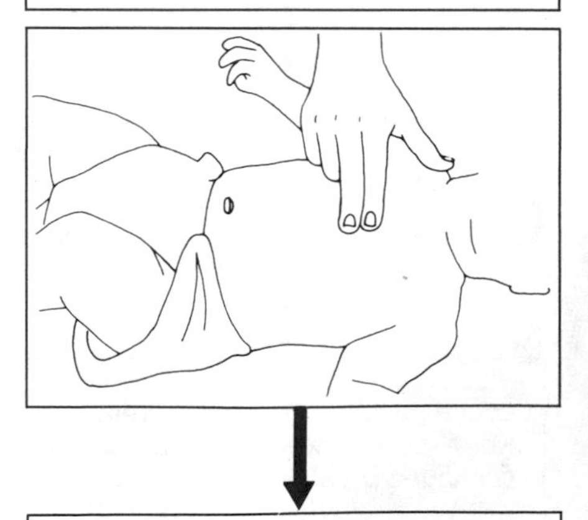

The compression/relaxation combination is performed at a rate of 120 times per minute. Count 1-2-3, etc.

Although the necessary fundamentals for performing CPR are set forth on this chart, there is no substitute for a course in CPR given by a certified instructor.

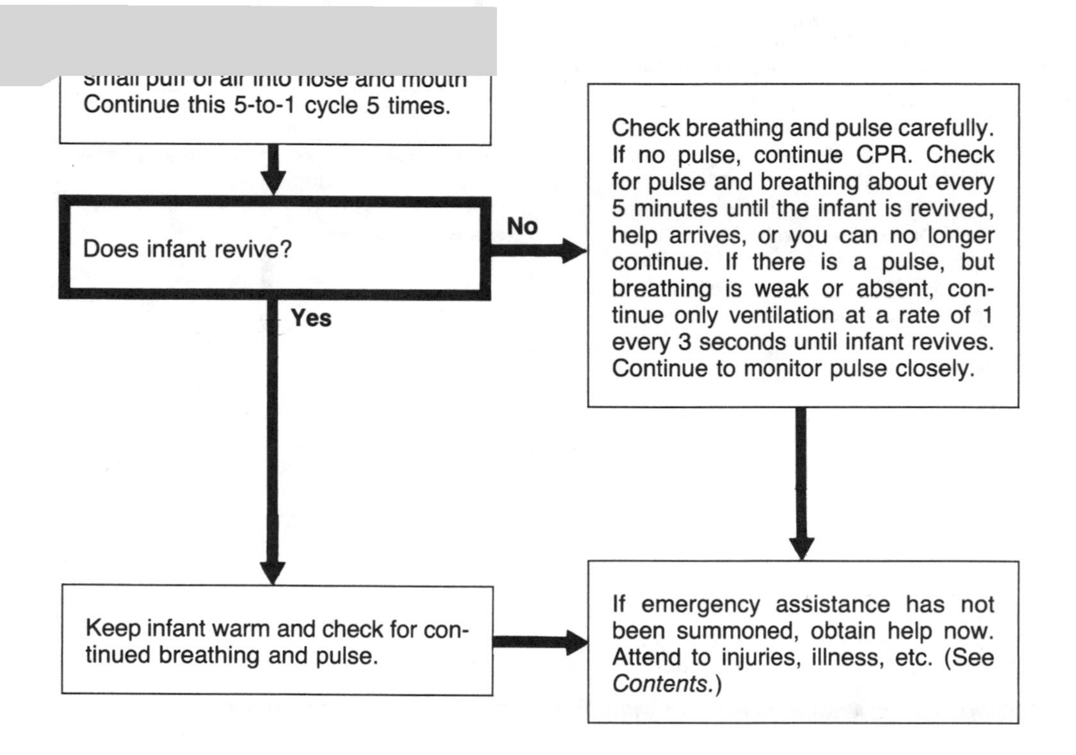
Continue this 5-to-1 cycle 5 times.
Does infant revive?
No
Yes
Check breathing and pulse carefully. If no pulse, continue CPR. Check for pulse and breathing about every 5 minutes until the infant is revived, help arrives, or you can no longer continue. If there is a pulse, but breathing is weak or absent, continue only ventilation at a rate of 1 every 3 seconds until infant revives. Continue to monitor pulse closely.
Keep infant warm and check for continued breathing and pulse.
If emergency assistance has not been summoned, obtain help now. Attend to injuries, illness, etc. (See *Contents*.)

*If neck is injured and you are trained in CPR, use the jaw thrust maneuver.

8 Childbirth
(Delivery)

Do not try to slow or speed delivery. Do not let the woman cross her legs or go to the bathroom. Do not place anything into the birth canal. Once you decide there is not enough time to reach the hospital, call for emergency assistance and a physician, or, if impossible, someone who has assisted in childbirth. Follow the procedures outlined below while awaiting assistance.

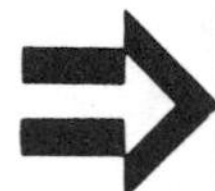

Cover a hard bed, or, if the woman cannot get to a bed, a long, sturdy table, the floor, or car seat with a thick layer of newspaper and, on hard surfaces, blankets. Cover this with clean sheets. Help the woman remove clothes and underclothes and have her lie on her back on the covered surface, with legs spread apart, knees bent, and feet flat. Place a folded blanket covered with a clean towel under her buttocks. During a contraction, observe the birth canal (the vagina).

Is any part of the baby besides the head (for example, buttocks, umbilical cord, arm, leg, or shoulder) visible?

No

Cover the woman's stomach with a clean sheet. If vomiting occurs turn the head to side and wipe mouth with tissue- or gauze-wrapped finger.

Assemble the following materials:
—a heavy plastic bag or shallow bowl,
—a new razor blade or, if unavailable, a pair of rust-free scissors,
—three new white shoelaces or strips of clean sheeting,
—several sanitary napkins,
—sterile gauze or clean cloth,
—a warm baby blanket or towel,
—aluminium foil.

Wash your hands thoroughly. Put scissors, if new razor blade is not available, and shoelaces or cloth strips into a pan or hot water. Ideally, they should be boiled for 20 minutes. Boil them as long as possible up to 20 minutes and allow time for cooling on sterile gauze or clean cloth before they are needed. Meanwhile, continue with the delivery.

Yes

Help the woman put on a robe, coat, or jacket. If the umbilical cord is protruding from the vagina:
—Have the woman remain in a knee-to-chest position and keep her legs from pinching the cord.
—Wash your hands thoroughly.
—Put your hand on baby's head and push it back into the vagina away from the cord.
—Cover cord with a clean towel.

Wait for assistance and obtain further instructions by phone from physician or hospital. (If in a car, drive to the hospital or physician's office as quickly—but safely—as possible.)

Calm the woman by talking while attending to the problem. Explain what you are doing. Try not to show anxiety; act with confidence. Your calm behavior can help to reassure the woman.

If childbirth is imminent while driving, follow these procedures as closely as possible; do not worry if some materials are not available.

As the baby's head emerges, guide and support the baby's head through the birth canal, keeping it free of blood and fluid. Do not pull or twist the head, but exert just enough pressure to keep it from popping out suddenly. If the baby is still inside the bag of waters, tear the bag open to prevent suffocation. The baby's head may be face down and, upon emerging, may turn to the side. If it does not, do not be alarmed.

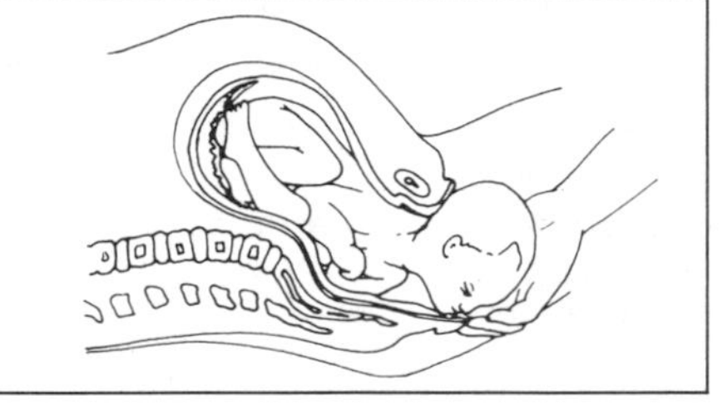

Is the umbilical cord around the infant's neck?

No / **Yes**

Yes: *If the cord is looped only once,* gently slip your finger between it and the baby's neck, then slip the cord over the head. *If this is impossible, or if the cord is looped more than once,* tie and knot the shoelaces or cloth strips around the cord, 2 inches apart. Carefully cut the cord between the knots with the sterile scissors and loosen the cord from the baby's neck.

No (and after the Yes step): Using a finger wrapped in gauze or clean cloth, gently wipe out the baby's mouth, still supporting, but not turning, the head. Do not wipe the ears, eyes, or nose, and do not wipe off the film on the baby's body.

When the baby's shoulders begin to emerge, lift the head and shoulders slightly while the body emerges. Support the baby under the armpits; be careful—do not let it slip.

See *Childbirth (Immediately After Delivery),* p. 9.

9 Childbirth
(Immediately After Delivery)

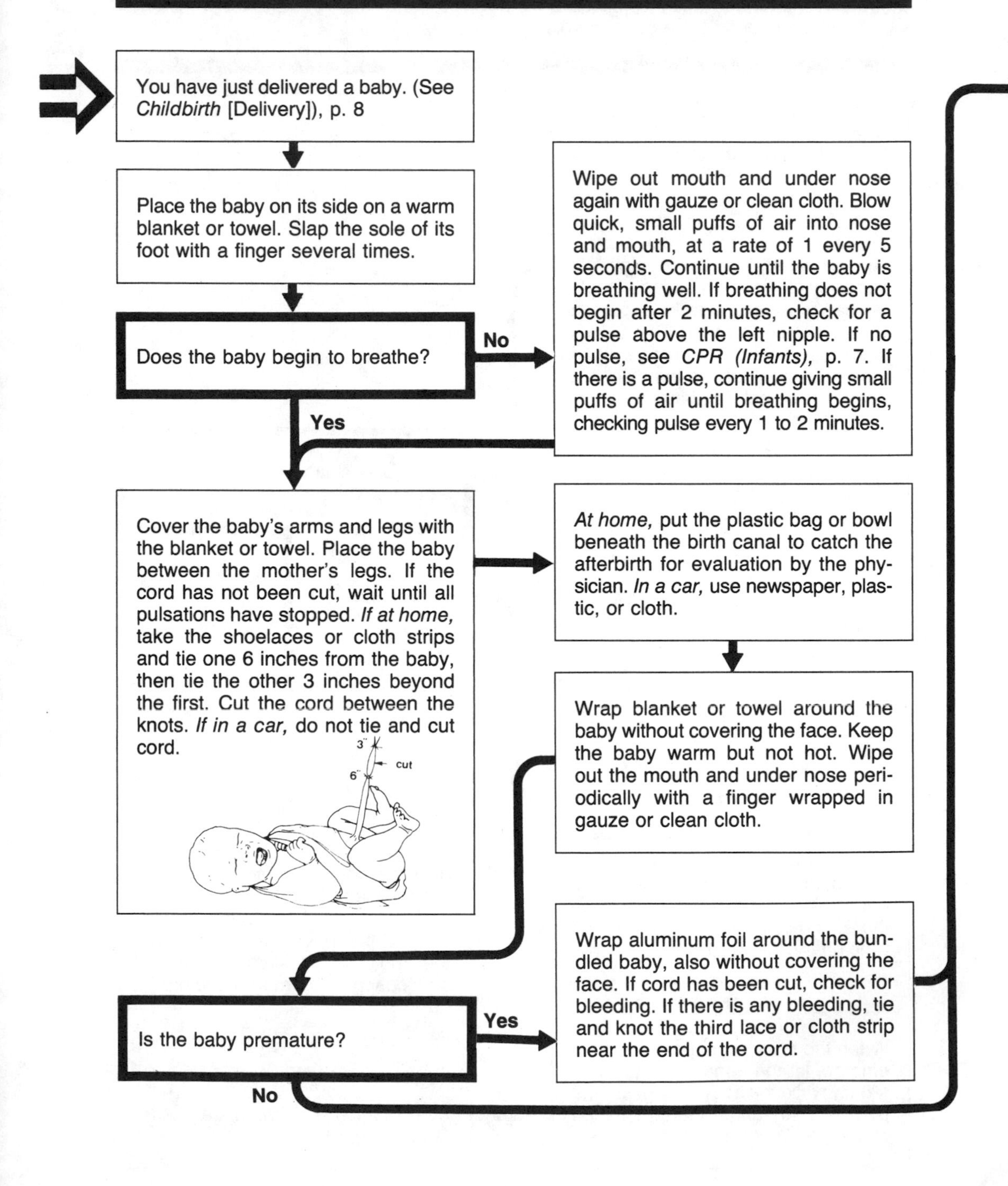

You have just delivered a baby. (See Childbirth [Delivery]), p. 8
Place the baby on its side on a warm blanket or towel. Slap the sole of its foot with a finger several times.
Does the baby begin to breathe?
No
Wipe out mouth and under nose again with gauze or clean cloth. Blow quick, small puffs of air into nose and mouth, at a rate of 1 every 5 seconds. Continue until the baby is breathing well. If breathing does not begin after 2 minutes, check for a pulse above the left nipple. If no pulse, see CPR (Infants), p. 7. If there is a pulse, continue giving small puffs of air until breathing begins, checking pulse every 1 to 2 minutes.
Yes
Cover the baby's arms and legs with the blanket or towel. Place the baby between the mother's legs. If the cord has not been cut, wait until all pulsations have stopped. If at home, take the shoelaces or cloth strips and tie one 6 inches from the baby, then tie the other 3 inches beyond the first. Cut the cord between the knots. If in a car, do not tie and cut cord.
3"
cut
6"
At home, put the plastic bag or bowl beneath the birth canal to catch the afterbirth for evaluation by the physician. In a car, use newspaper, plastic, or cloth.
Wrap blanket or towel around the baby without covering the face. Keep the baby warm but not hot. Wipe out the mouth and under nose periodically with a finger wrapped in gauze or clean cloth.
Is the baby premature?
Yes
Wrap aluminum foil around the bundled baby, also without covering the face. If cord has been cut, check for bleeding. If there is any bleeding, tie and knot the third lace or cloth strip near the end of the cord.
No

Calm the woman by talking while attending to the problem. Explain what you are doing. Try not to show anxiety; act with confidence. Your calm behavior can help to reassure the woman.

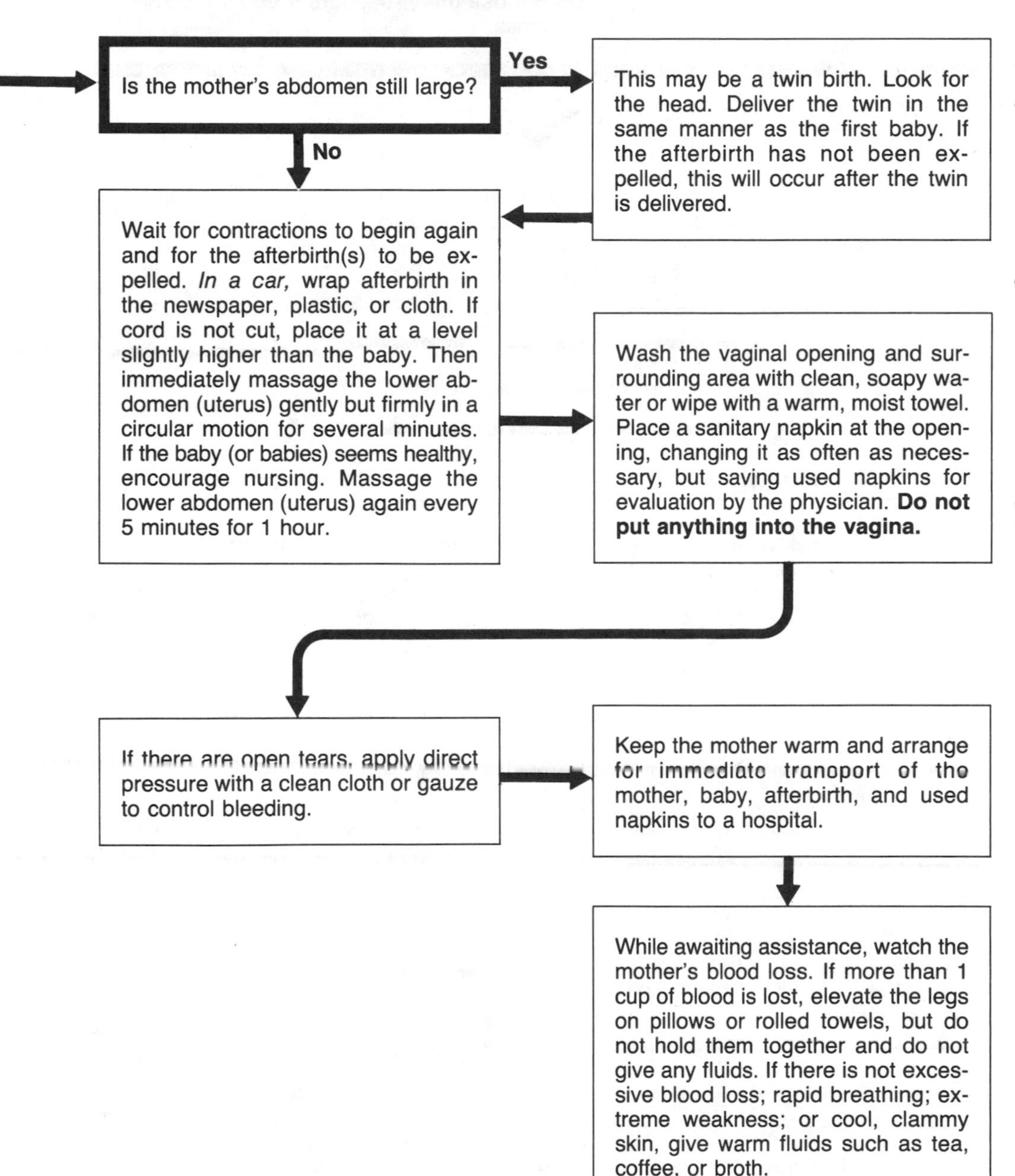
Is the mother's abdomen still large?
Yes
This may be a twin birth. Look for the head. Deliver the twin in the same manner as the first baby. If the afterbirth has not been expelled, this will occur after the twin is delivered.
No
Wait for contractions to begin again and for the afterbirth(s) to be expelled. In a car, wrap afterbirth in the newspaper, plastic, or cloth. If cord is not cut, place it at a level slightly higher than the baby. Then immediately massage the lower abdomen (uterus) gently but firmly in a circular motion for several minutes. If the baby (or babies) seems healthy, encourage nursing. Massage the lower abdomen (uterus) again every 5 minutes for 1 hour.
Wash the vaginal opening and surrounding area with clean, soapy water or wipe with a warm, moist towel. Place a sanitary napkin at the opening, changing it as often as necessary, but saving used napkins for evaluation by the physician. Do not put anything into the vagina.
If there are open tears, apply direct pressure with a clean cloth or gauze to control bleeding.
Keep the mother warm and arrange for immediate transport of the mother, baby, afterbirth, and used napkins to a hospital.
While awaiting assistance, watch the mother's blood loss. If more than 1 cup of blood is lost, elevate the legs on pillows or rolled towels, but do not hold them together and do not give any fluids. If there is not excessive blood loss; rapid breathing; extreme weakness; or cool, clammy skin, give warm fluids such as tea, coffee, or broth.

10 Choking

Signs & Symptoms: *Clutching throat/initial coughing with gasping followed by inability to cough, speak, or breathe/sudden loss of consciousness while eating/blue or gray skin, fingernails, and mucous membranes.*

Do not use this procedure if person is able to speak.

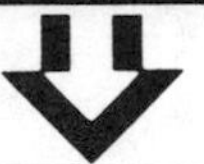

If the person has been injured, do not move unless necessary. Use appropriate method shown below to dislodge obstruction.

The person who is choking is:

Infant

Hold infant face down, supporting head. Deliver 4 back blows with the heel of your hand between infant's shoulder blades. Repeat if necessary.

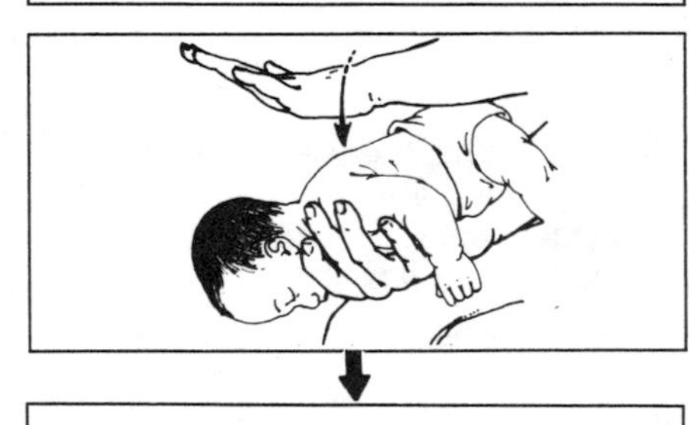

If object has not been dislodged, obtain emergency assistance. If dislodged, seek medical care immediately

Small Child

Place child face up on your lap. Place your index and middle fingers above child's navel but below the rib cage and quickly but gently thrust in and up. Repeat several times if necessary

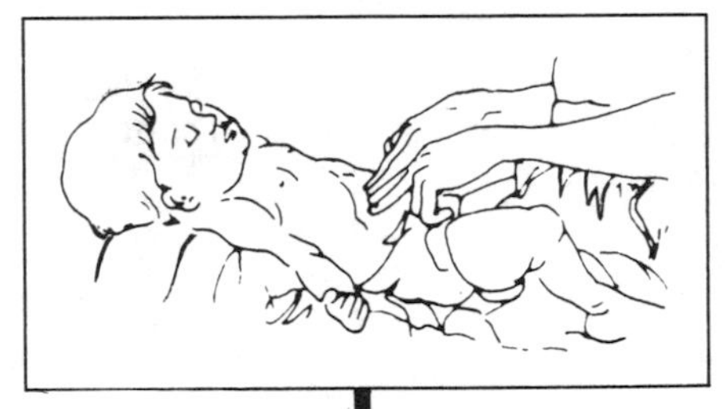

Has object been dislodged?

Yes

Have the child checked by a physician immediately.*

No

Turn child upside down and deliver 4 sharp blows between shoulder blades. Repeat if necessary. If still not dislodged, obtain emergency assistance. If dislodged, seek medical care immediately.*

If person was not eating, clutches chest, or indicates there is extreme chest pain, see *Chest Pain,* p. 13.
Shout for help even if you think you are alone. If there are two or more rescuers, one should obtain emergency assistance while the other is following the procedures outlined below.

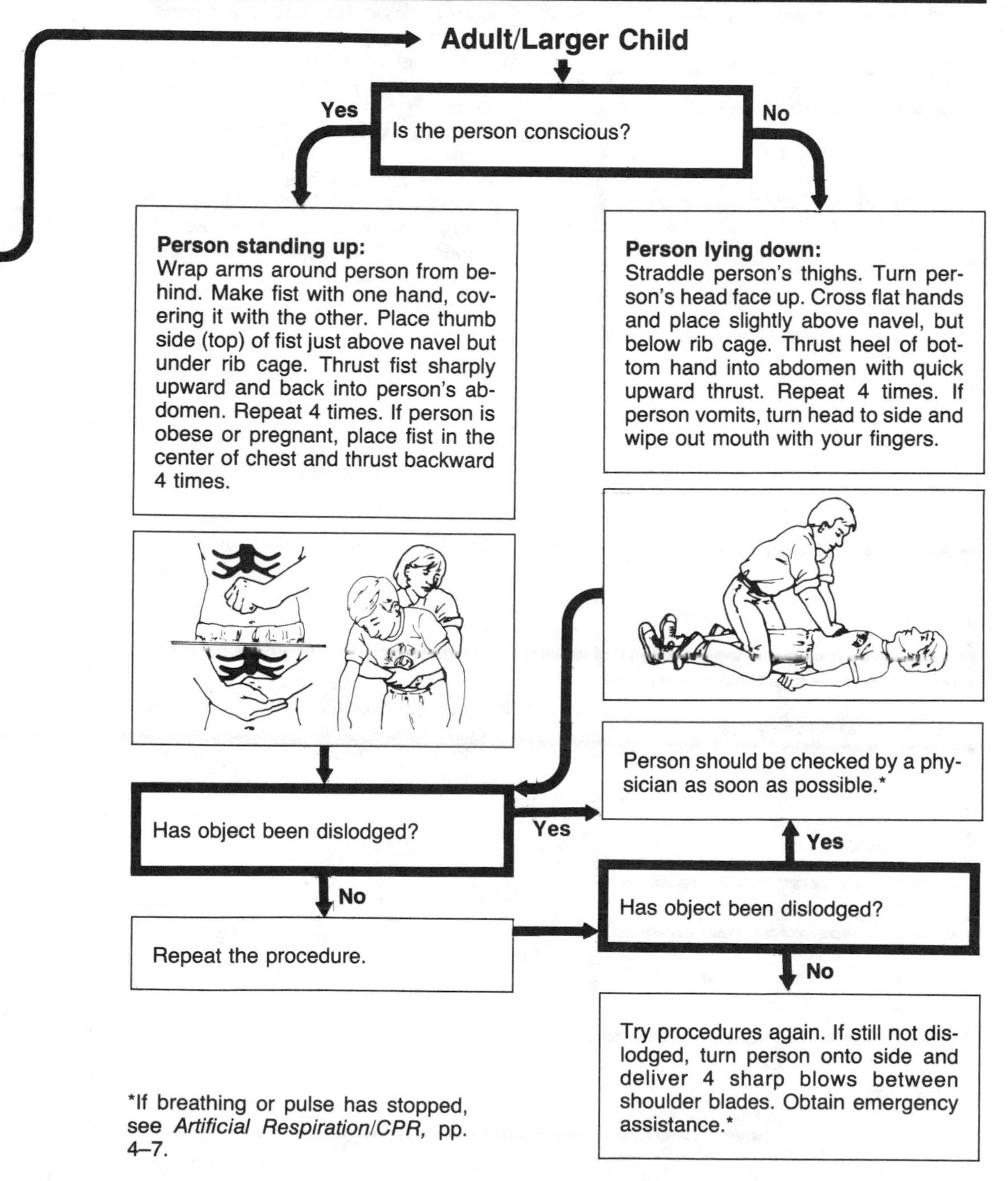
Adult/Larger Child
Is the person conscious?
Yes
No
Person standing up:
Wrap arms around person from behind. Make fist with one hand, covering it with the other. Place thumb side (top) of fist just above navel but under rib cage. Thrust fist sharply upward and back into person's abdomen. Repeat 4 times. If person is obese or pregnant, place fist in the center of chest and thrust backward 4 times.
Person lying down:
Straddle person's thighs. Turn person's head face up. Cross flat hands and place slightly above navel, but below rib cage. Thrust heel of bottom hand into abdomen with quick upward thrust. Repeat 4 times. If person vomits, turn head to side and wipe out mouth with your fingers.
Has object been dislodged?
Yes
Person should be checked by a physician as soon as possible.*
No
Repeat the procedure.
Has object been dislodged?
Yes
No
Try procedures again. If still not dislodged, turn person onto side and deliver 4 sharp blows between shoulder blades. Obtain emergency assistance.*

*If breathing or pulse has stopped, see *Artificial Respiration/CPR,* pp. 4–7.

11 Abdominal Pain

Abdominal pain should never be taken lightly. Keep person lying quietly. Do not apply heat to abdomen.

If you suspect *Chemical Poisoning,* see p. 32.

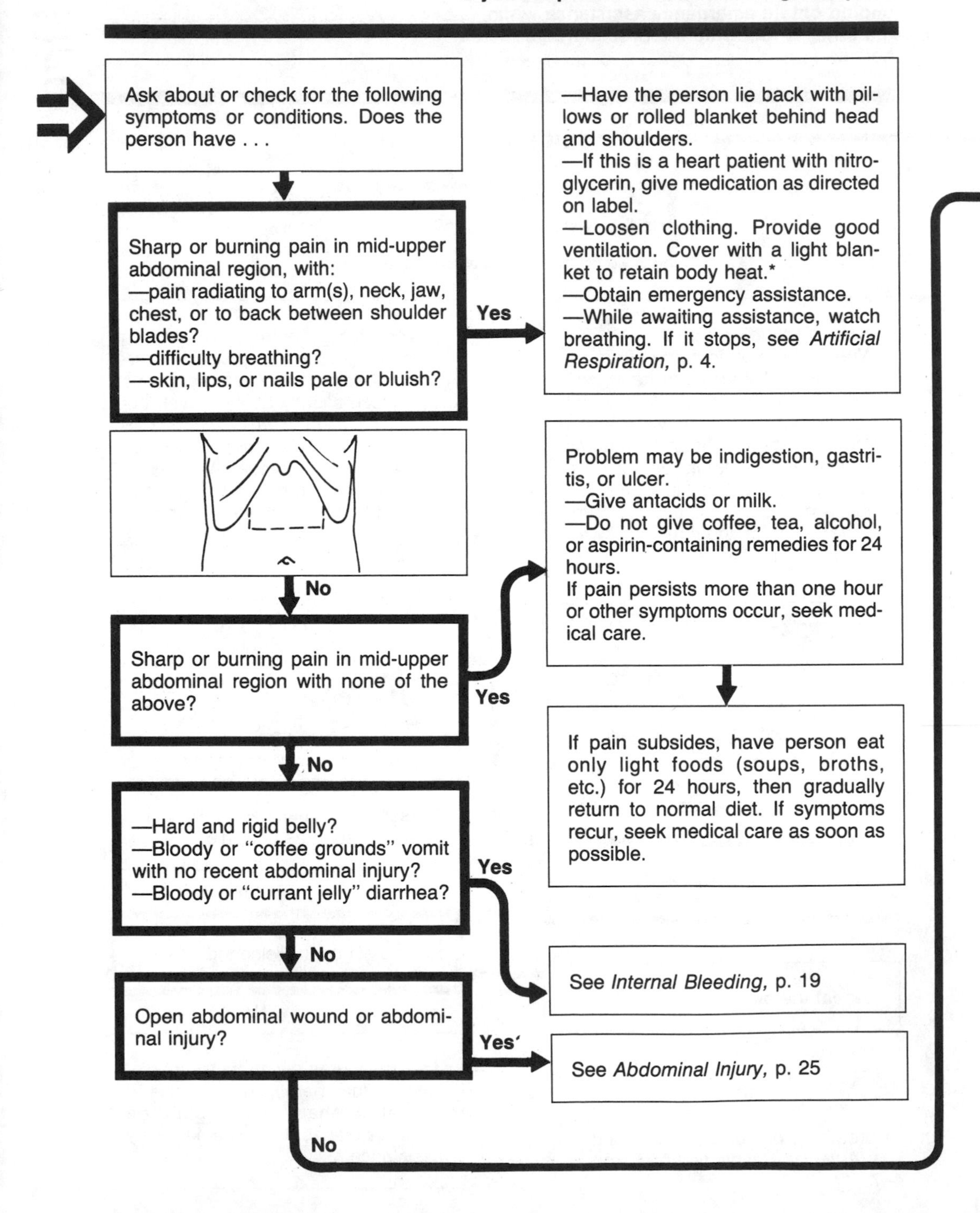

Ask about or check for the following symptoms or conditions. Does the person have . . .
Sharp or burning pain in mid-upper abdominal region, with:
—pain radiating to arm(s), neck, jaw, chest, or to back between shoulder blades?
—difficulty breathing?
—skin, lips, or nails pale or bluish?
Yes
—Have the person lie back with pillows or rolled blanket behind head and shoulders.
—If this is a heart patient with nitroglycerin, give medication as directed on label.
—Loosen clothing. Provide good ventilation. Cover with a light blanket to retain body heat.*
—Obtain emergency assistance.
—While awaiting assistance, watch breathing. If it stops, see Artificial Respiration, p. 4.
No
Sharp or burning pain in mid-upper abdominal region with none of the above?
Yes
Problem may be indigestion, gastritis, or ulcer.
—Give antacids or milk.
—Do not give coffee, tea, alcohol, or aspirin-containing remedies for 24 hours.
If pain persists more than one hour or other symptoms occur, seek medical care.
If pain subsides, have person eat only light foods (soups, broths, etc.) for 24 hours, then gradually return to normal diet. If symptoms recur, seek medical care as soon as possible.
No
—Hard and rigid belly?
—Bloody or "coffee grounds" vomit with no recent abdominal injury?
—Bloody or "currant jelly" diarrhea?
Yes
See Internal Bleeding, p. 19
No
Open abdominal wound or abdominal injury?
Yes
See Abdominal Injury, p. 25
No

Calm the person by talking while attending to the problem. Explain what you are doing. Try not to show anxiety; act with confidence. Your calm behavior can help to reassure the sick person.

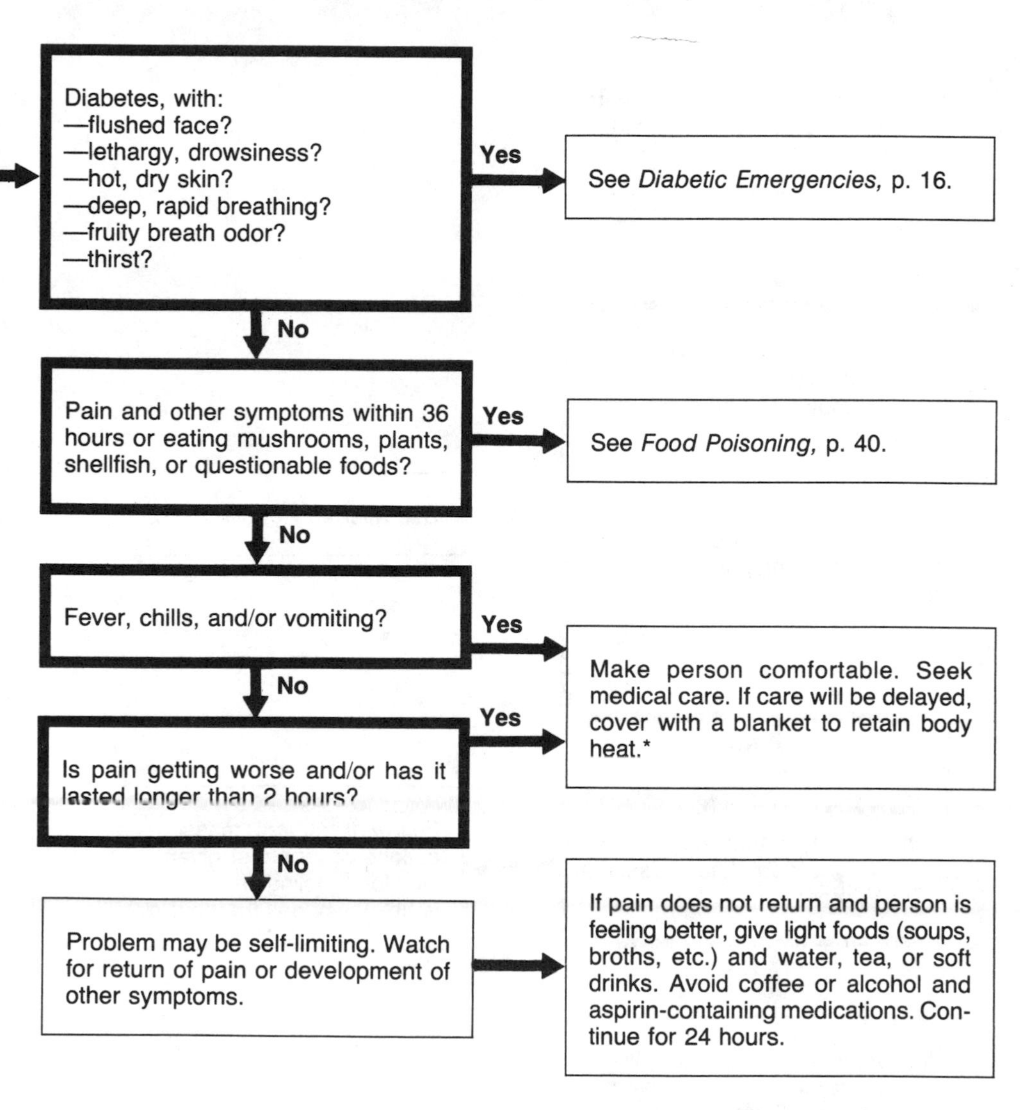
Diabetes, with:
—flushed face?
—lethargy, drowsiness?
—hot, dry skin?
—deep, rapid breathing?
—fruity breath odor?
—thirst?
Yes
See Diabetic Emergencies, p. 16.
No
Pain and other symptoms within 36 hours or eating mushrooms, plants, shellfish, or questionable foods?
Yes
See Food Poisoning, p. 40.
No
Fever, chills, and/or vomiting?
Yes
Make person comfortable. Seek medical care. If care will be delayed, cover with a blanket to retain body heat.*
No
Yes
Is pain getting worse and/or has it lasted longer than 2 hours?
No
Problem may be self-limiting. Watch for return of pain or development of other symptoms.
If pain does not return and person is feeling better, give light foods (soups, broths, etc.) and water, tea, or soft drinks. Avoid coffee or alcohol and aspirin-containing medications. Continue for 24 hours.

*If weather is very warm and person's skin does not feel cool and clammy, covering will not be necessary.

 # Asthma Attack

Signs & Symptoms: *wheezing/difficulty breathing/exhaling much more difficult than inhaling/rapid heartbeat/possible hard, tight cough/possible nasal congestion/possible pale, bluish skin, lips, and nails*

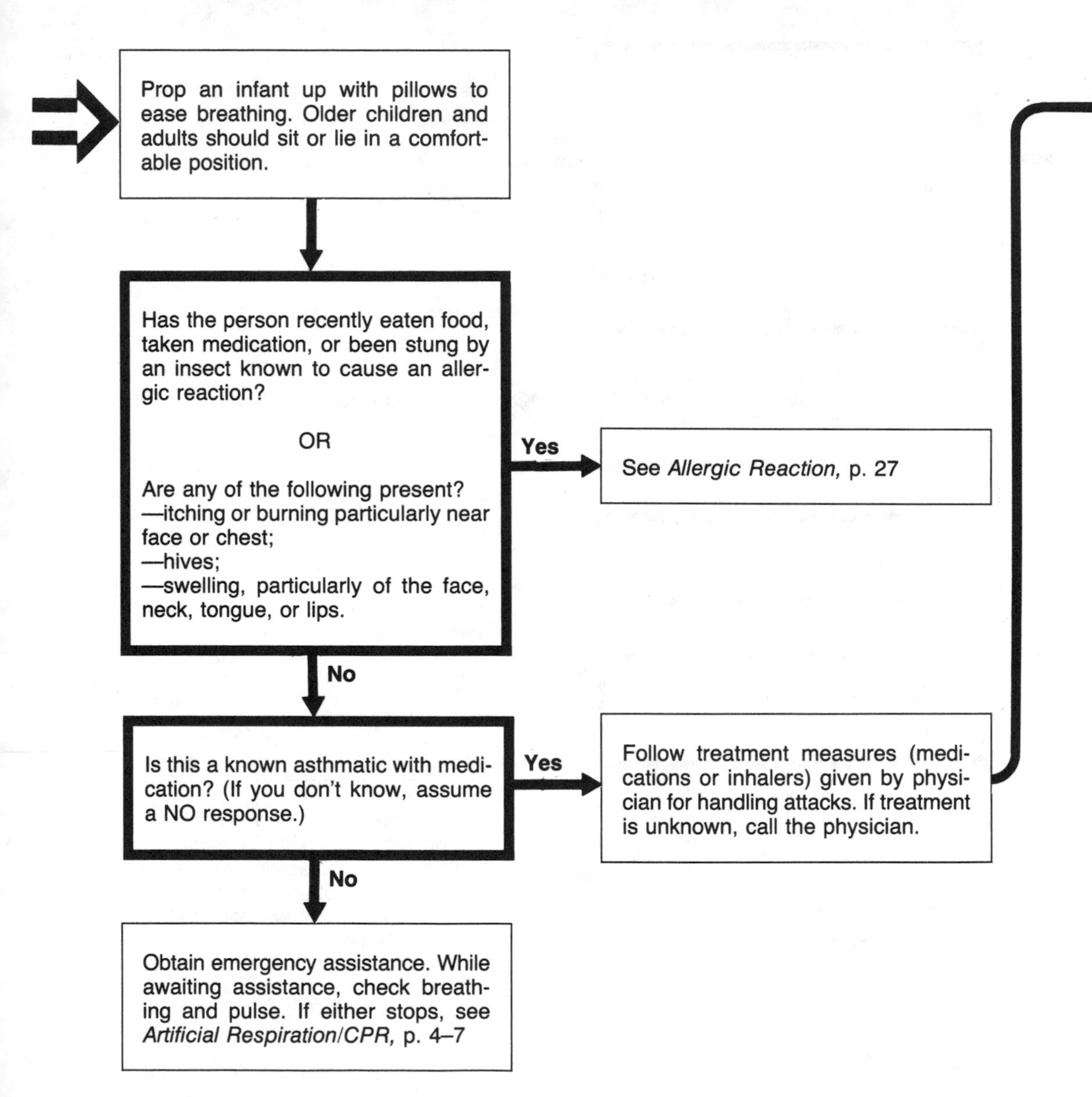

Prop an infant up with pillows to ease breathing. Older children and adults should sit or lie in a comfortable position.
Has the person recently eaten food, taken medication, or been stung by an insect known to cause an allergic reaction?
OR
Are any of the following present?
—itching or burning particularly near face or chest;
—hives;
—swelling, particularly of the face, neck, tongue, or lips.
Yes
See *Allergic Reaction,* p. 27
No
Is this a known asthmatic with medication? (If you don't know, assume a NO response.)
Yes
Follow treatment measures (medications or inhalers) given by physician for handling attacks. If treatment is unknown, call the physician.
No
Obtain emergency assistance. While awaiting assistance, check breathing and pulse. If either stops, see *Artificial Respiration/CPR,* p. 4–7

Calm the person by talking while attending to the problem. Explain what you are doing. Try not to show anxiety; act with confidence. Your calm behavior can help to reassure the sick person.

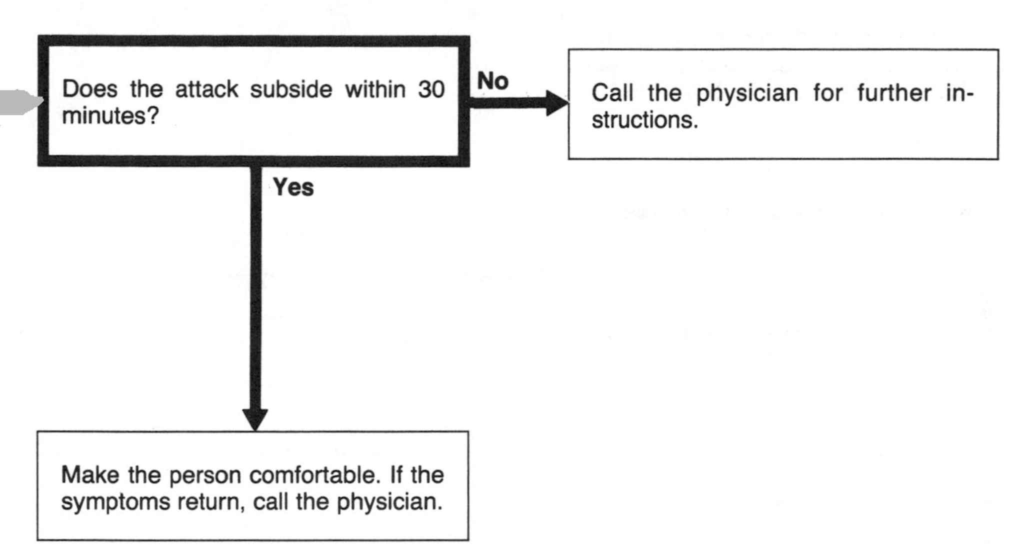
Does the attack subside within 30 minutes?
No
Call the physician for further instructions.
Yes
Make the person comfortable. If the symptoms return, call the physician.

13 Chest Pain

Most chest pain is caused by indigestion or muscular strain; however, check symptoms below for more serious ailments. Chest pain in a male over 25 or a female over 30 may indicate a heart problem.

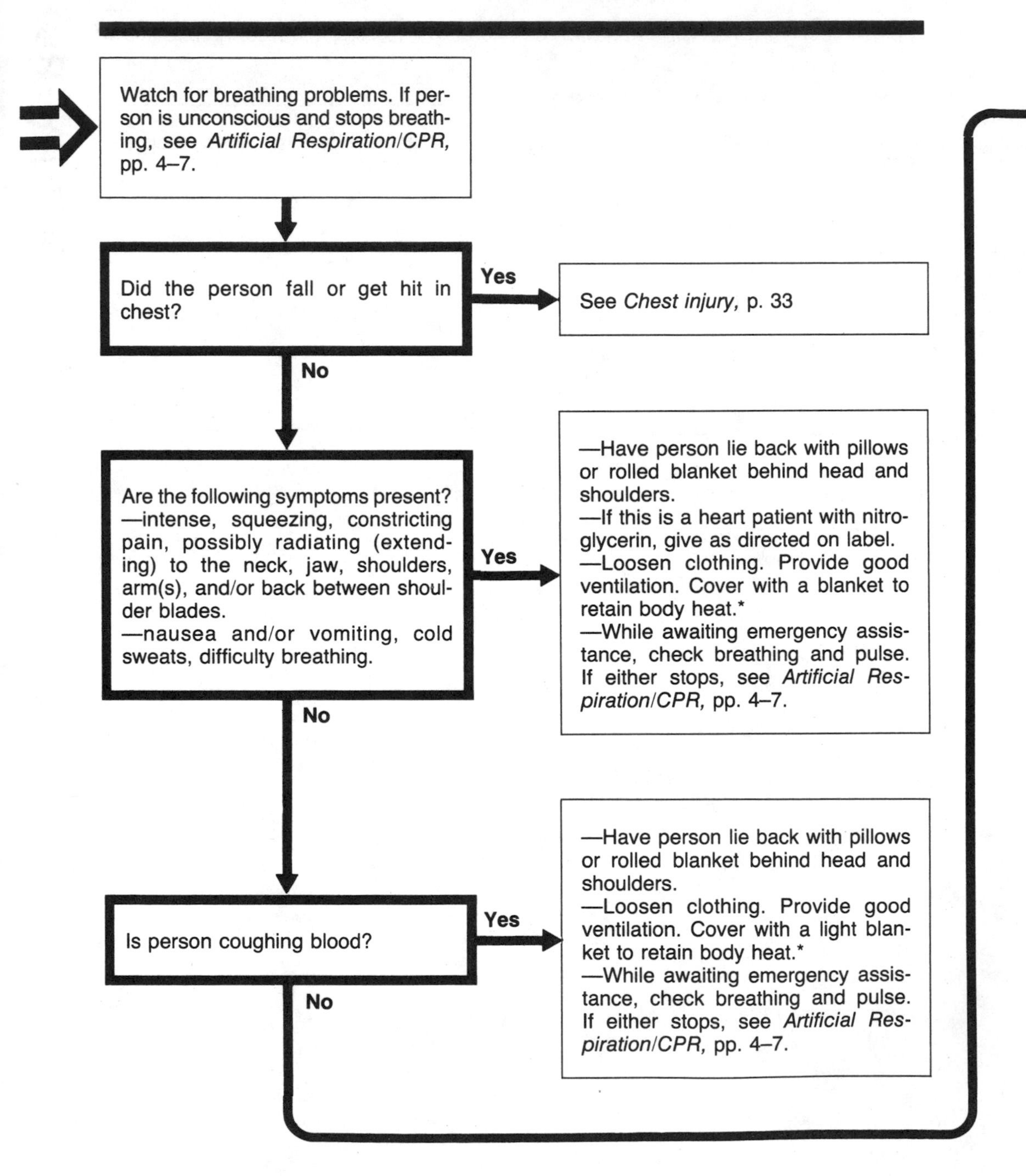

Watch for breathing problems. If person is unconscious and stops breathing, see *Artificial Respiration/CPR,* pp. 4–7.
Did the person fall or get hit in chest?
Yes
See *Chest injury,* p. 33
No
Are the following symptoms present?
—intense, squeezing, constricting pain, possibly radiating (extending) to the neck, jaw, shoulders, arm(s), and/or back between shoulder blades.
—nausea and/or vomiting, cold sweats, difficulty breathing.
Yes
—Have person lie back with pillows or rolled blanket behind head and shoulders.
—If this is a heart patient with nitroglycerin, give as directed on label.
—Loosen clothing. Provide good ventilation. Cover with a blanket to retain body heat.*
—While awaiting emergency assistance, check breathing and pulse. If either stops, see *Artificial Respiration/CPR,* pp. 4–7.
No
Is person coughing blood?
Yes
—Have person lie back with pillows or rolled blanket behind head and shoulders.
—Loosen clothing. Provide good ventilation. Cover with a light blanket to retain body heat.*
—While awaiting emergency assistance, check breathing and pulse. If either stops, see *Artificial Respiration/CPR,* pp. 4–7.
No

Calm the person by talking while attending to the problem. Explain what you are doing. Try not to show anxiety; act with confidence. Your calm behavior can help to reassure the sick person.

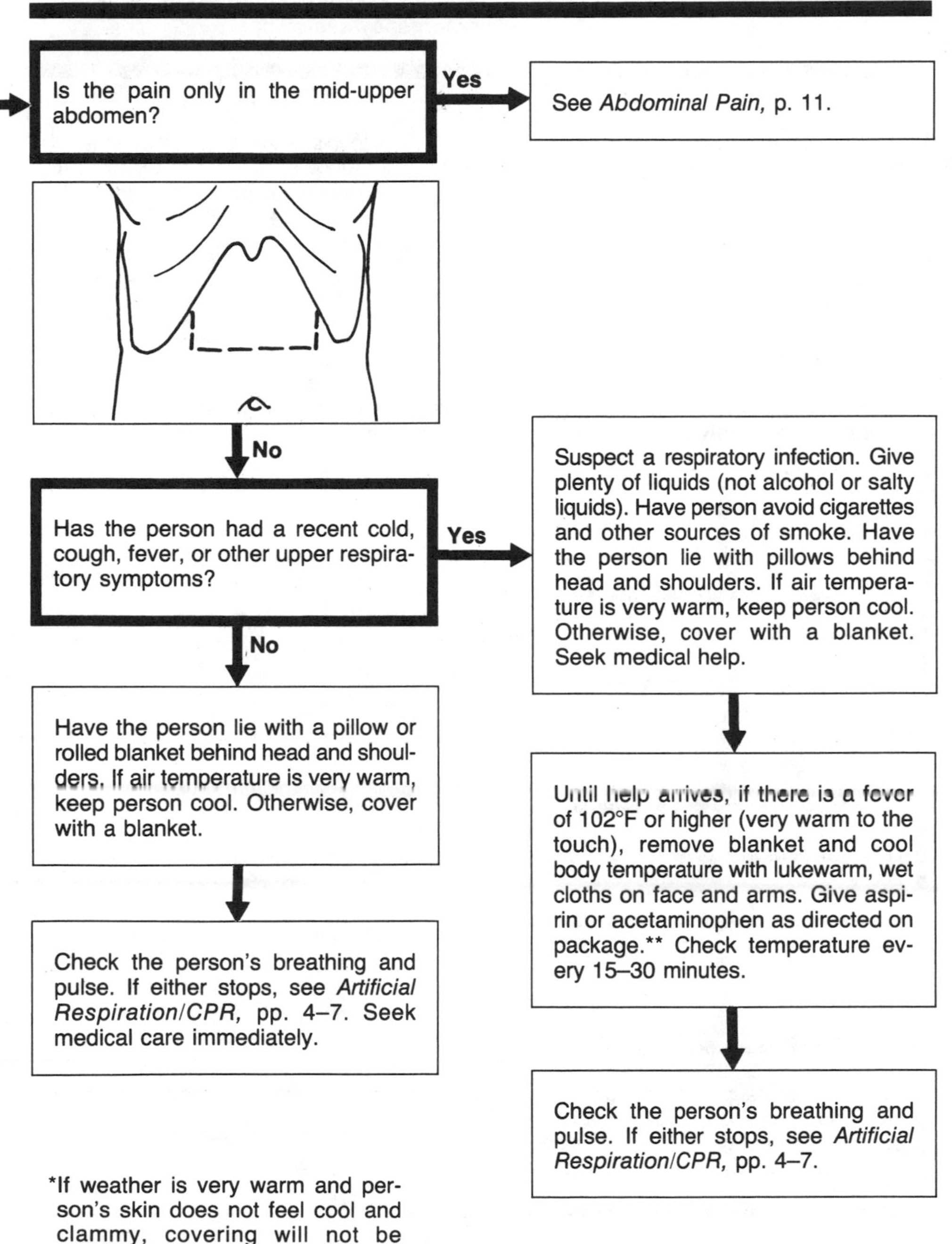

Is the pain only in the mid-upper abdomen?
Yes
See *Abdominal Pain,* p. 11.
No
Has the person had a recent cold, cough, fever, or other upper respiratory symptoms?
Yes
Suspect a respiratory infection. Give plenty of liquids (not alcohol or salty liquids). Have person avoid cigarettes and other sources of smoke. Have the person lie with pillows behind head and shoulders. If air temperature is very warm, keep person cool. Otherwise, cover with a blanket. Seek medical help.
Until help arrives, if there is a fever of 102°F or higher (very warm to the touch), remove blanket and cool body temperature with lukewarm, wet cloths on face and arms. Give aspirin or acetaminophen as directed on package.** Check temperature every 15–30 minutes.
Check the person's breathing and pulse. If either stops, see *Artificial Respiration/CPR,* pp. 4–7.
No
Have the person lie with a pillow or rolled blanket behind head and shoulders. If air temperature is very warm, keep person cool. Otherwise, cover with a blanket.
Check the person's breathing and pulse. If either stops, see *Artificial Respiration/CPR,* pp. 4–7. Seek medical care immediately.

*If weather is very warm and person's skin does not feel cool and clammy, covering will not be necessary.

**Do not give aspirin to a child with the flu.

Convulsion

(Including Epileptic Seizure)

Signs & Symptoms: *involuntary jerking of muscles/possible loss of bowel and bladder control/unconsciousness/cessation of breathing/gradual subsidence followed by semiconsciousness*

For any convulsions or seizures, obtain emergency assistance.

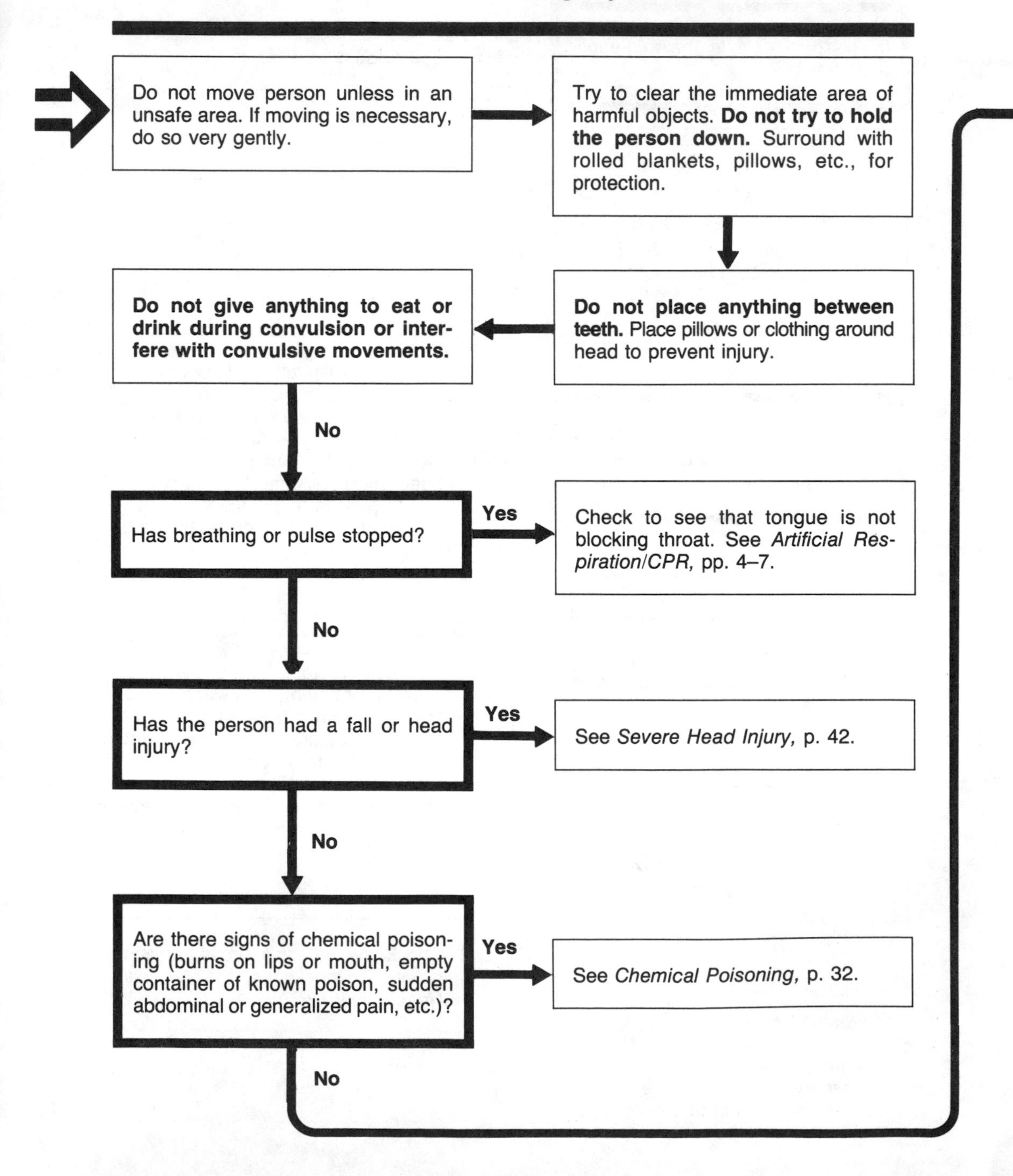
Do not move person unless in an unsafe area. If moving is necessary, do so very gently.
Try to clear the immediate area of harmful objects. **Do not try to hold the person down.** Surround with rolled blankets, pillows, etc., for protection.
Do not place anything between teeth. Place pillows or clothing around head to prevent injury.
Do not give anything to eat or drink during convulsion or interfere with convulsive movements.
No
Has breathing or pulse stopped?
Yes
Check to see that tongue is not blocking throat. See *Artificial Respiration/CPR,* pp. 4–7.
No
Has the person had a fall or head injury?
Yes
See *Severe Head Injury,* p. 42.
No
Are there signs of chemical poisoning (burns on lips or mouth, empty container of known poison, sudden abdominal or generalized pain, etc.)?
Yes
See *Chemical Poisoning,* p. 32.
No

Calm the person by talking while attending to the problem. Explain what you are doing. Try not to show anxiety; act with confidence. Your calm behavior can help to reassure the sick or injured person.

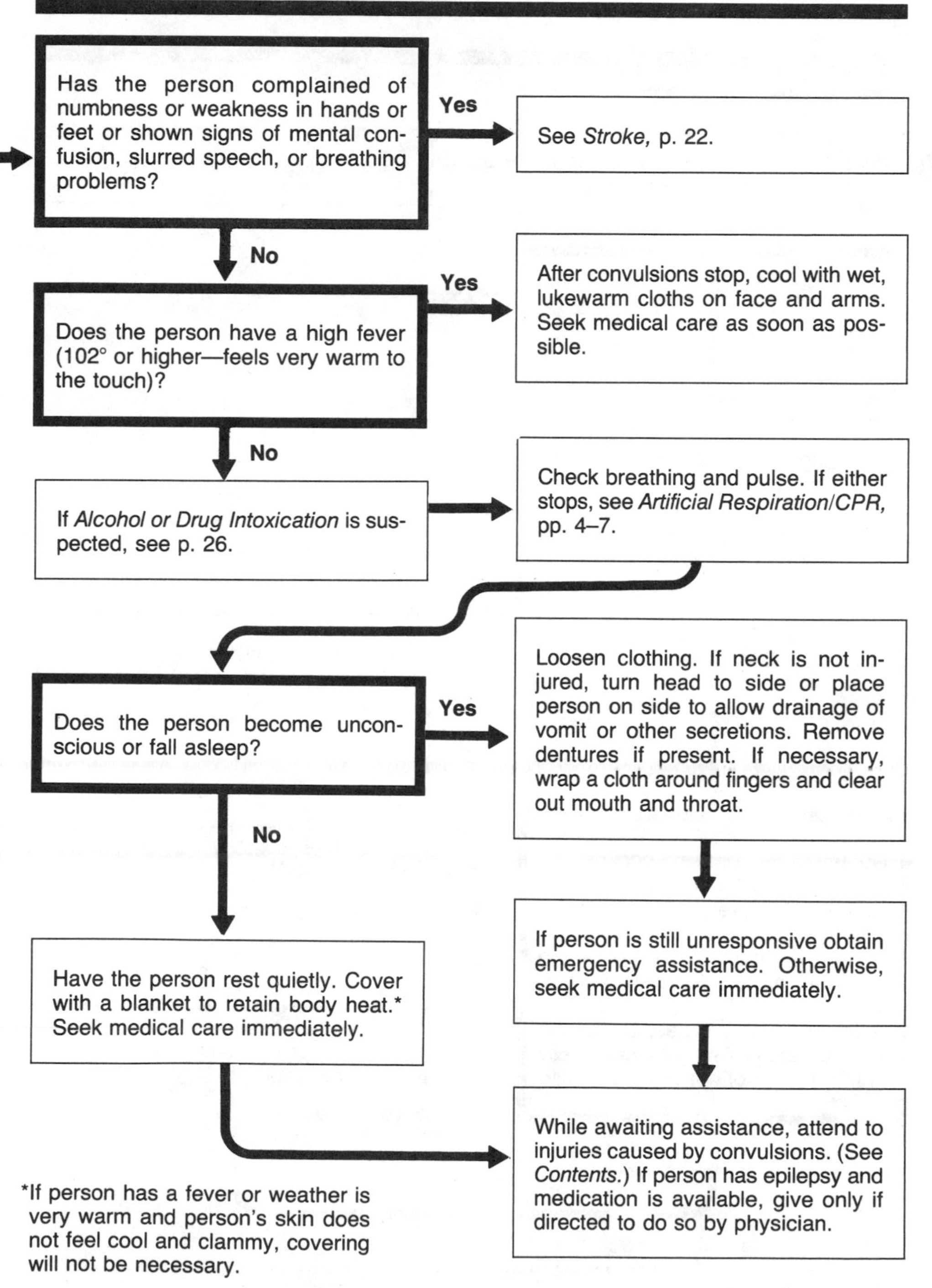
Has the person complained of numbness or weakness in hands or feet or shown signs of mental confusion, slurred speech, or breathing problems?
Yes
See Stroke, p. 22.
No
Does the person have a high fever (102° or higher—feels very warm to the touch)?
Yes
After convulsions stop, cool with wet, lukewarm cloths on face and arms. Seek medical care as soon as possible.
No
If Alcohol or Drug Intoxication is suspected, see p. 26.
Check breathing and pulse. If either stops, see Artificial Respiration/CPR, pp. 4–7.
Does the person become unconscious or fall asleep?
Yes
Loosen clothing. If neck is not injured, turn head to side or place person on side to allow drainage of vomit or other secretions. Remove dentures if present. If necessary, wrap a cloth around fingers and clear out mouth and throat.
If person is still unresponsive obtain emergency assistance. Otherwise, seek medical care immediately.
No
Have the person rest quietly. Cover with a blanket to retain body heat.*
Seek medical care immediately.
While awaiting assistance, attend to injuries caused by convulsions. (See Contents.) If person has epilepsy and medication is available, give only if directed to do so by physician.

*If person has a fever or weather is very warm and person's skin does not feel cool and clammy, covering will not be necessary.

15 Croup Attack

Signs & Symptoms: *barklike, ringing cough/very difficult inhalation/possible difficulty exhaling/spasms or involuntary muscle contractions of the larynx (voice box)/tight, painful chest muscles/recent cold or upper respiratory infection/rapid pulse/possible fever/possible pale, bluish lips and nails.*

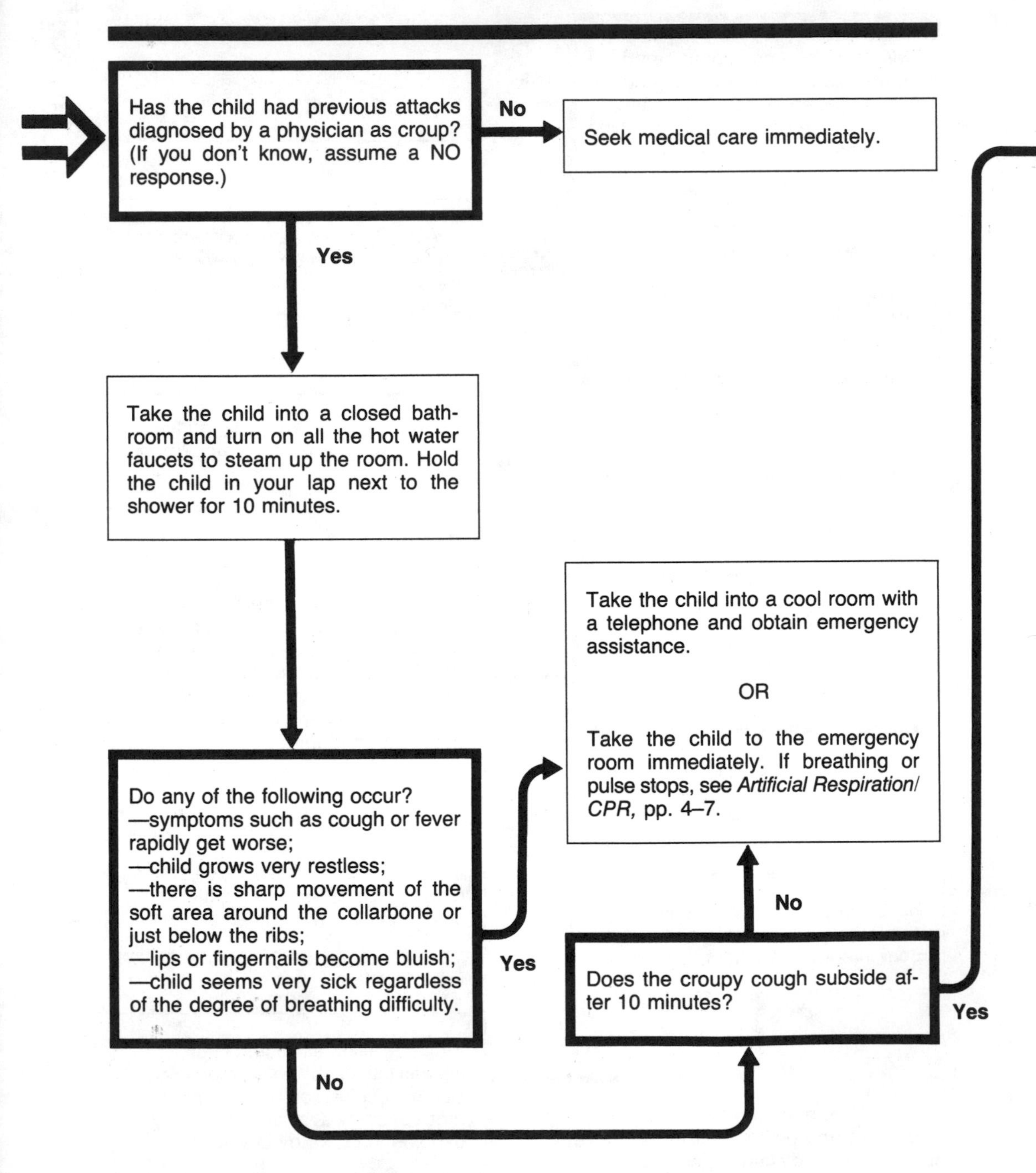

Has the child had previous attacks diagnosed by a physician as croup? (If you don't know, assume a NO response.)
No
Seek medical care immediately.
Yes
Take the child into a closed bathroom and turn on all the hot water faucets to steam up the room. Hold the child in your lap next to the shower for 10 minutes.
Do any of the following occur?
—symptoms such as cough or fever rapidly get worse;
—child grows very restless;
—there is sharp movement of the soft area around the collarbone or just below the ribs;
—lips or fingernails become bluish;
—child seems very sick regardless of the degree of breathing difficulty.
Yes
Take the child into a cool room with a telephone and obtain emergency assistance.
OR
Take the child to the emergency room immediately. If breathing or pulse stops, see Artificial Respiration/CPR, pp. 4–7.
No
No
Does the croupy cough subside after 10 minutes?
Yes

Calm the person by talking while attending to the problem. Explain what you are doing. Try not to show anxiety, act with confidence. Your calm behavior can help to reassure the sick person.

If your child has a severe croup attack while traveling, seek medical care.

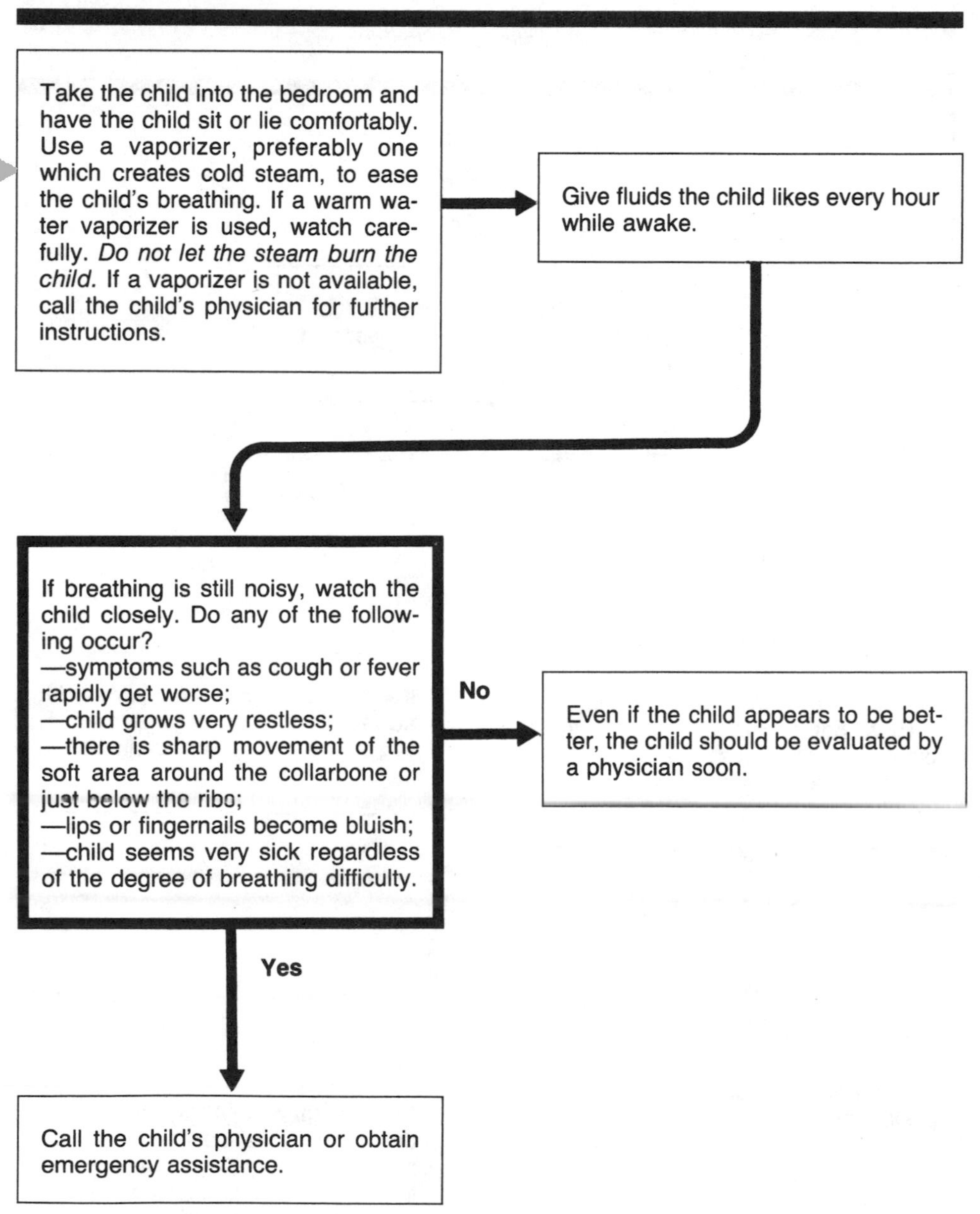
Take the child into the bedroom and have the child sit or lie comfortably. Use a vaporizer, preferably one which creates cold steam, to ease the child's breathing. If a warm water vaporizer is used, watch carefully. *Do not let the steam burn the child.* If a vaporizer is not available, call the child's physician for further instructions.
Give fluids the child likes every hour while awake.
If breathing is still noisy, watch the child closely. Do any of the following occur?
—symptoms such as cough or fever rapidly get worse;
—child grows very restless;
—there is sharp movement of the soft area around the collarbone or just below the ribs;
—lips or fingernails become bluish;
—child seems very sick regardless of the degree of breathing difficulty.
No
Even if the child appears to be better, the child should be evaluated by a physician soon.
Yes
Call the child's physician or obtain emergency assistance.

16 Diabetic Emergencies

Signs & Symptoms:
Uncontrolled diabetes (early warning): *flushed face/dry skin/fruity breath odor/headache/thirst/drowsiness/ nausea/rapid pulse/rapid breathing/possible abdominal pain or vomiting*
Insulin shock (early warning): *hunger/weakness/shakiness/faintness/heavy sweating/blurred vision/rapid pulse/cool and clammy skin/anxiety/restlessness/confusion*

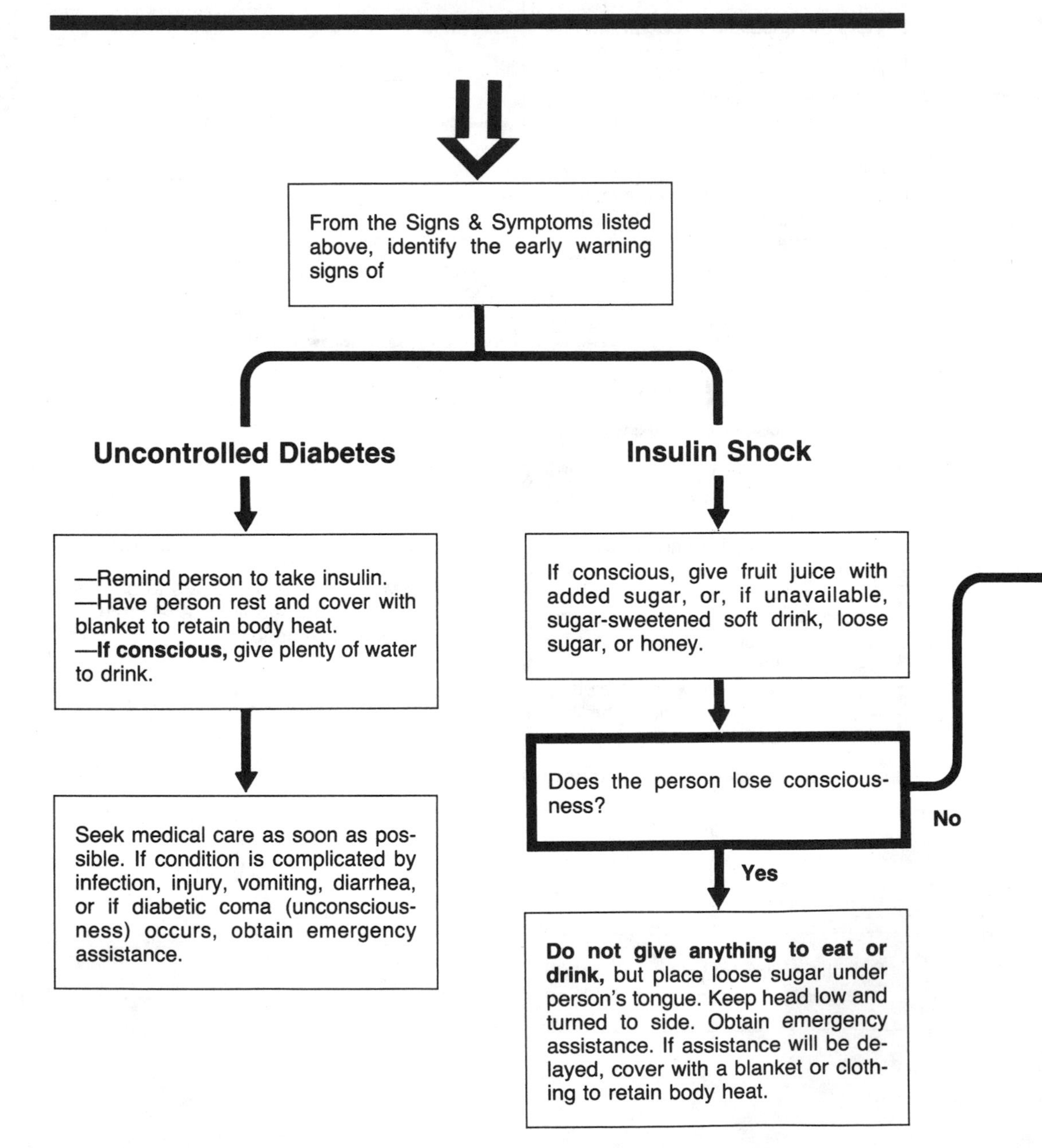

From the Signs & Symptoms listed above, identify the early warning signs of
Uncontrolled Diabetes
—Remind person to take insulin.
—Have person rest and cover with blanket to retain body heat.
—If conscious, give plenty of water to drink.
Seek medical care as soon as possible. If condition is complicated by infection, injury, vomiting, diarrhea, or if diabetic coma (unconsciousness) occurs, obtain emergency assistance.
Insulin Shock
If conscious, give fruit juice with added sugar, or, if unavailable, sugar-sweetened soft drink, loose sugar, or honey.
Does the person lose consciousness?
No
Yes
Do not give anything to eat or drink, but place loose sugar under person's tongue. Keep head low and turned to side. Obtain emergency assistance. If assistance will be delayed, cover with a blanket or clothing to retain body heat.

Calm the person by talking while attending to the problem. Explain what you are doing. Try not to show anxiety; act with confidence. Your calm behavior can help to reassure the sick person.

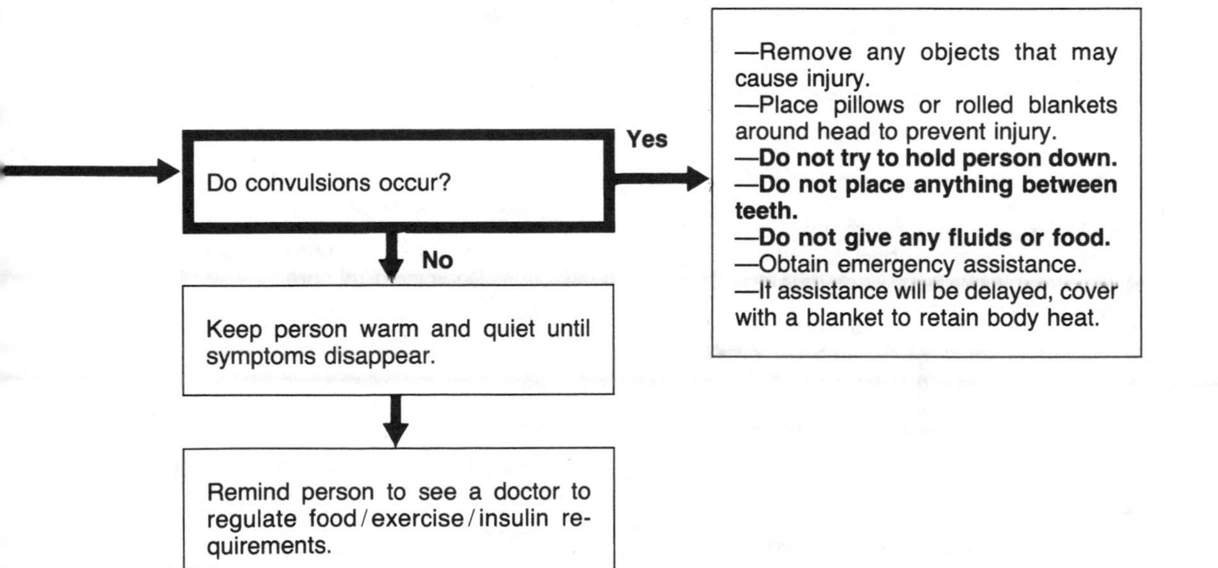
Do convulsions occur?
Yes
—Remove any objects that may cause injury.
—Place pillows or rolled blankets around head to prevent injury.
—Do not try to hold person down.
—Do not place anything between teeth.
—Do not give any fluids or food.
—Obtain emergency assistance.
—If assistance will be delayed, cover with a blanket to retain body heat.
No
Keep person warm and quiet until symptoms disappear.
Remind person to see a doctor to regulate food/exercise/insulin requirements.

17 Fever

Do not assume an extremely high temperature to be serious, or a low temperature to be insignificant. Look for additional signs & symptoms. (Example: children often react to minor problems with high temperatures. On the other hand, a serious problem such as meningitis often is accompanied by low fever—101°F.)

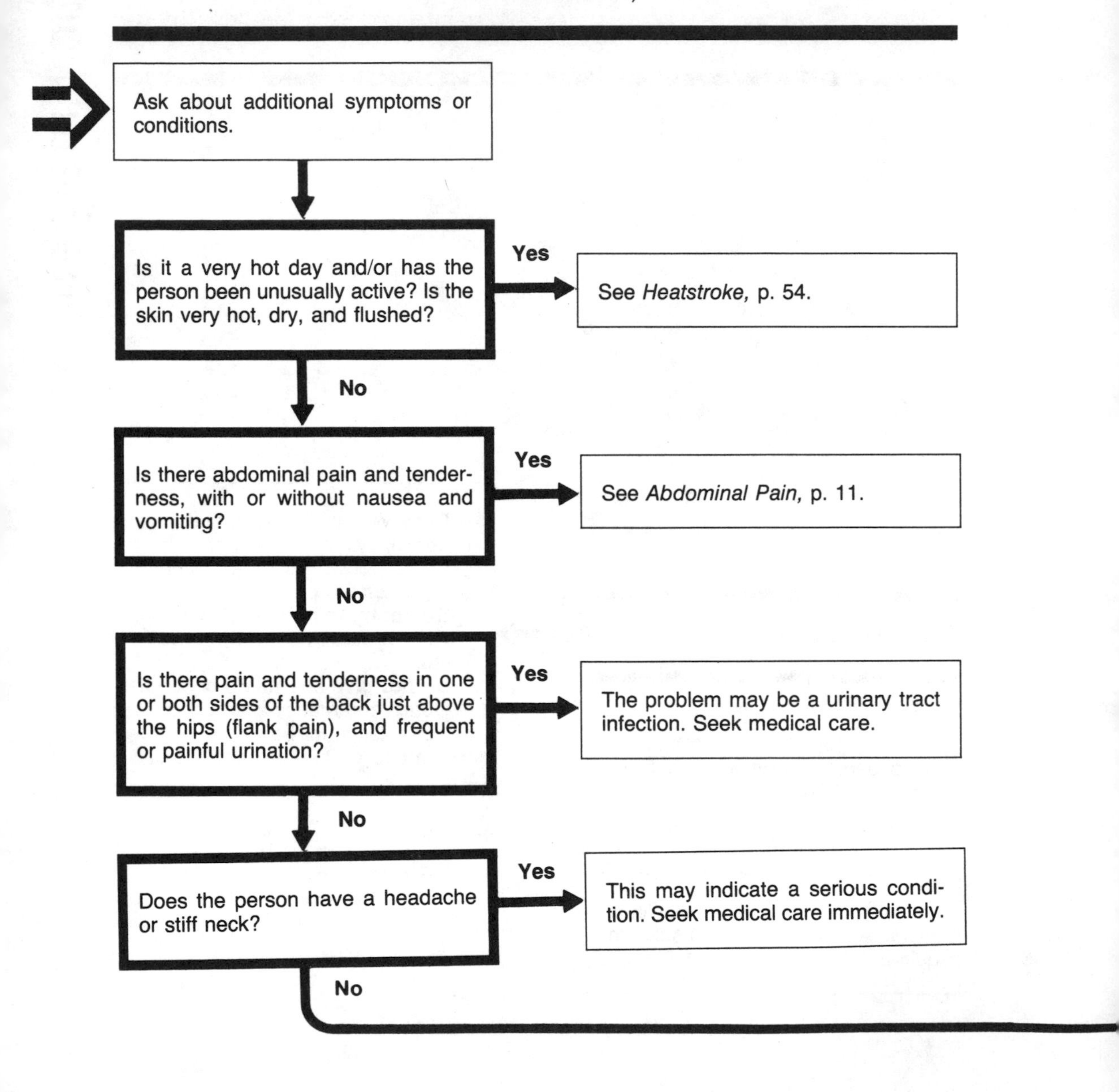

Ask about additional symptoms or conditions.
Is it a very hot day and/or has the person been unusually active? Is the skin very hot, dry, and flushed?
Yes
See *Heatstroke,* p. 54.
No
Is there abdominal pain and tenderness, with or without nausea and vomiting?
Yes
See *Abdominal Pain,* p. 11.
No
Is there pain and tenderness in one or both sides of the back just above the hips (flank pain), and frequent or painful urination?
Yes
The problem may be a urinary tract infection. Seek medical care.
No
Does the person have a headache or stiff neck?
Yes
This may indicate a serious condition. Seek medical care immediately.
No

Calm the person by talking while attending to the problem. Explain what you are doing. Try not to show anxiety; act with confidence. Your calm behavior can help to reassure the sick person.

Suspect a viral or bacterial infection, especially if the person has a sore throat, cough, muscle pain, chills, or has been in contact with someone with similar symptoms.

Have the person rest quietly. If fever is 102°F or higher (very warm to the touch), cool body temperature with lukewarm, wet cloths on face, arms, groin, and armpits. Give aspirin or acetaminophen as directed on package.* Given plenty of clear fluids if awake.

Watch for convulsions, especially in children. If these occur, see *Convulsion*, p. 14. Watch for: rapid breathing; cold, clammy skin; weakness. If these develop, cover person with a blanket and elevate legs with pillows or rolled blankets and obtain emergency assistance.

Contact a physician for further advice.

*Do not give aspirin to a child with the flu.

Headache

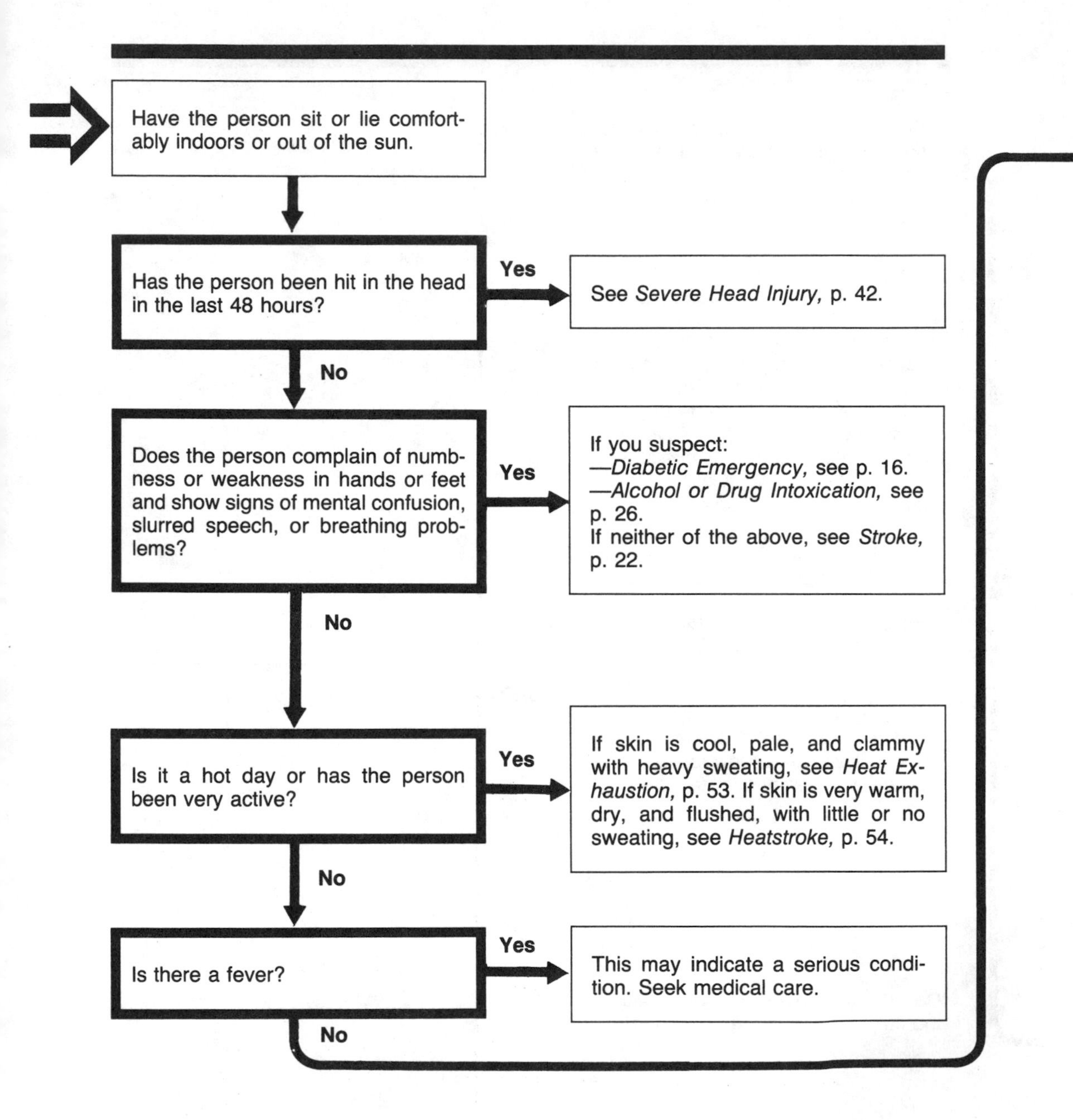

Have the person sit or lie comfortably indoors or out of the sun.
Has the person been hit in the head in the last 48 hours?
Yes
See *Severe Head Injury,* p. 42.
No
Does the person complain of numbness or weakness in hands or feet and show signs of mental confusion, slurred speech, or breathing problems?
Yes
If you suspect:
—*Diabetic Emergency,* see p. 16.
—*Alcohol or Drug Intoxication,* see p. 26.
If neither of the above, see *Stroke,* p. 22.
No
Is it a hot day or has the person been very active?
Yes
If skin is cool, pale, and clammy with heavy sweating, see *Heat Exhaustion,* p. 53. If skin is very warm, dry, and flushed, with little or no sweating, see *Heatstroke,* p. 54.
No
Is there a fever?
Yes
This may indicate a serious condition. Seek medical care.
No

Calm the person by talking while attending to the problem. Explain what you are doing. Try not to show anxiety; act with confidence. Your calm behavior can help to reassure the sick or injured person.

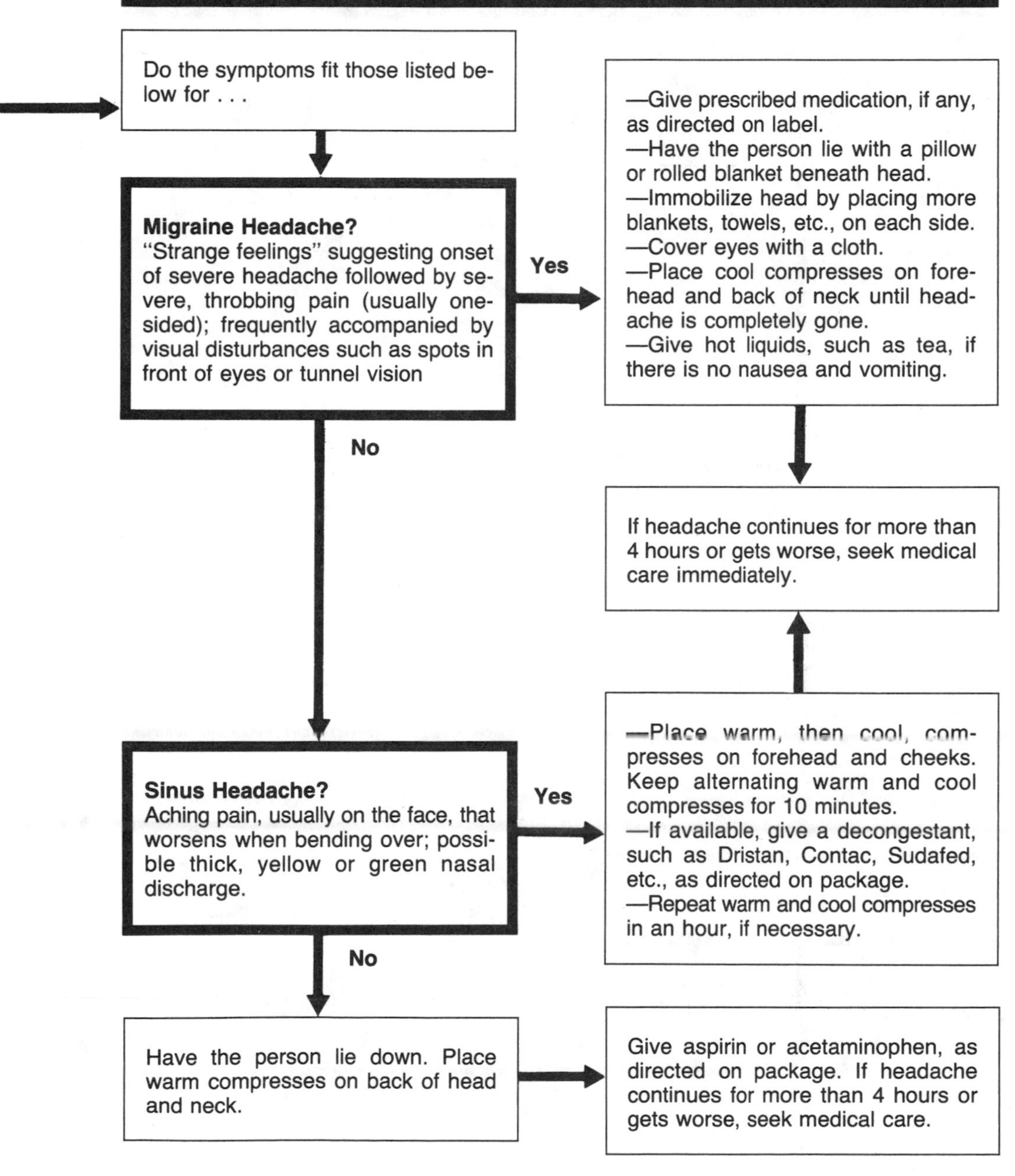
Do the symptoms fit those listed below for . . .
Migraine Headache?
"Strange feelings" suggesting onset of severe headache followed by severe, throbbing pain (usually one-sided); frequently accompanied by visual disturbances such as spots in front of eyes or tunnel vision
Yes
—Give prescribed medication, if any, as directed on label.
—Have the person lie with a pillow or rolled blanket beneath head.
—Immobilize head by placing more blankets, towels, etc., on each side.
—Cover eyes with a cloth.
—Place cool compresses on forehead and back of neck until headache is completely gone.
—Give hot liquids, such as tea, if there is no nausea and vomiting.
If headache continues for more than 4 hours or gets worse, seek medical care immediately.
No
Sinus Headache?
Aching pain, usually on the face, that worsens when bending over; possible thick, yellow or green nasal discharge.
Yes
—Place warm, then cool, compresses on forehead and cheeks. Keep alternating warm and cool compresses for 10 minutes.
—If available, give a decongestant, such as Dristan, Contac, Sudafed, etc., as directed on package.
—Repeat warm and cool compresses in an hour, if necessary.
No
Have the person lie down. Place warm compresses on back of head and neck.
Give aspirin or acetaminophen, as directed on package. If headache continues for more than 4 hours or gets worse, seek medical care.

19 Internal Bleeding or Infection

Possible Signs & Symptoms: *bloody or "coffee grounds" vomit/smoky or bloody urine/dark, bloody, or tarlike stools/pink or bloody sputum/ extreme paleness/weak or rapid pulse/cold, clammy skin/anxiety/thirst/rapid breathing/localized tenderness and swelling/rigid abdomen/abdominal pain/unconsciousness*

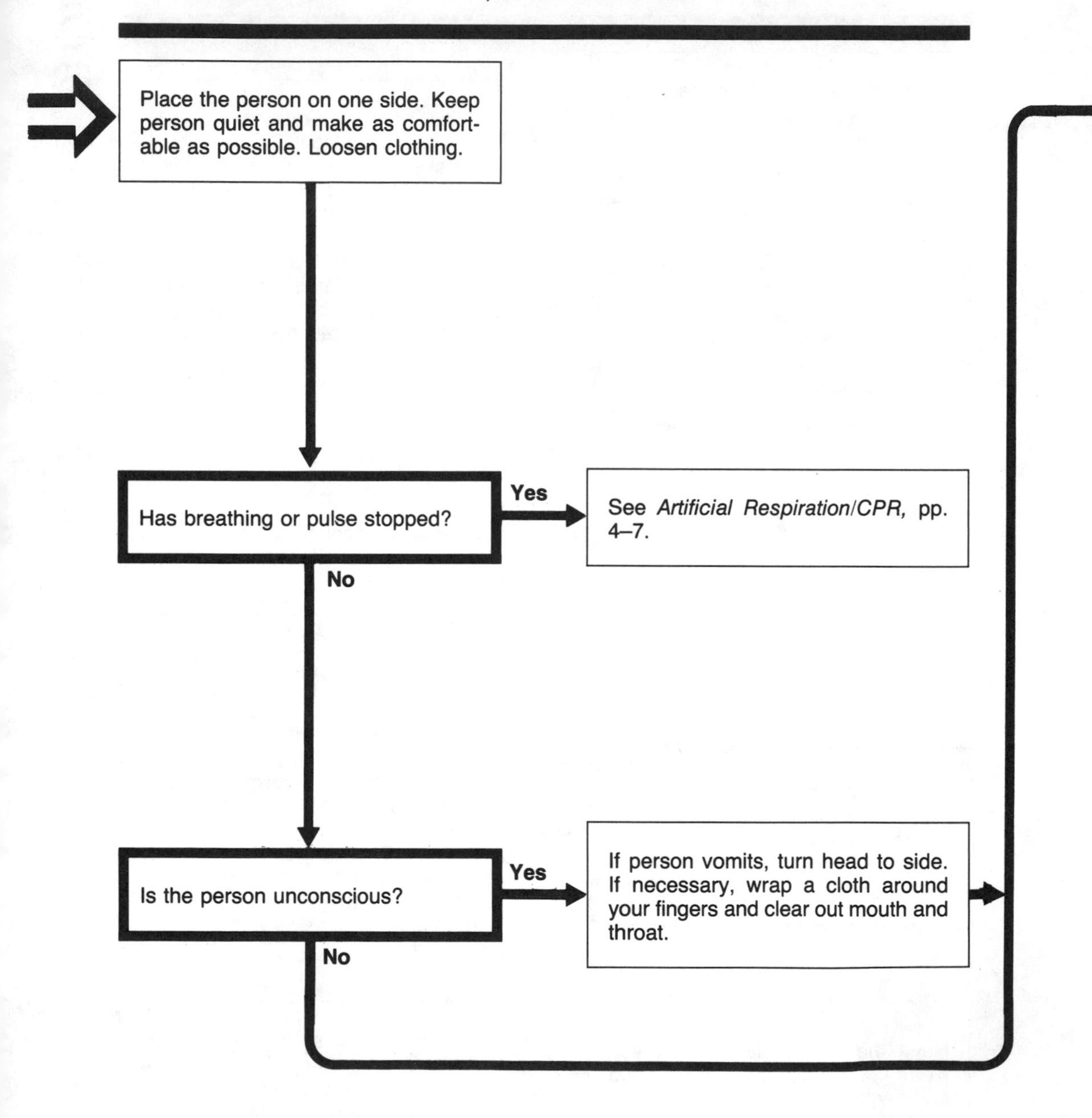

Place the person on one side. Keep person quiet and make as comfortable as possible. Loosen clothing.
Has breathing or pulse stopped?
Yes
See *Artificial Respiration/CPR,* pp. 4–7.
No
Is the person unconscious?
Yes
If person vomits, turn head to side. If necessary, wrap a cloth around your fingers and clear out mouth and throat.
No

Calm the person by talking while attending to the problem. Explain what you are doing. Try not to show anxiety; act with confidence. Your calm behavior can help to reassure the sick person.

If there are two or more rescuers, one should obtain emergency assistance while the other is following the procedures outlined below.

If emergency assistance has not been summoned, obtain help now. While awaiting assistance:
—**Do not give anything to eat or drink.**
—If person's skin feels cold and clammy, elevate legs on pillows and cover with a light blanket or clothing to retain body heat.
—Continue to check breathing and pulse. If either stops, see *Artificial Respiration/CPR,* pp. 4–7.

Nausea & Vomiting

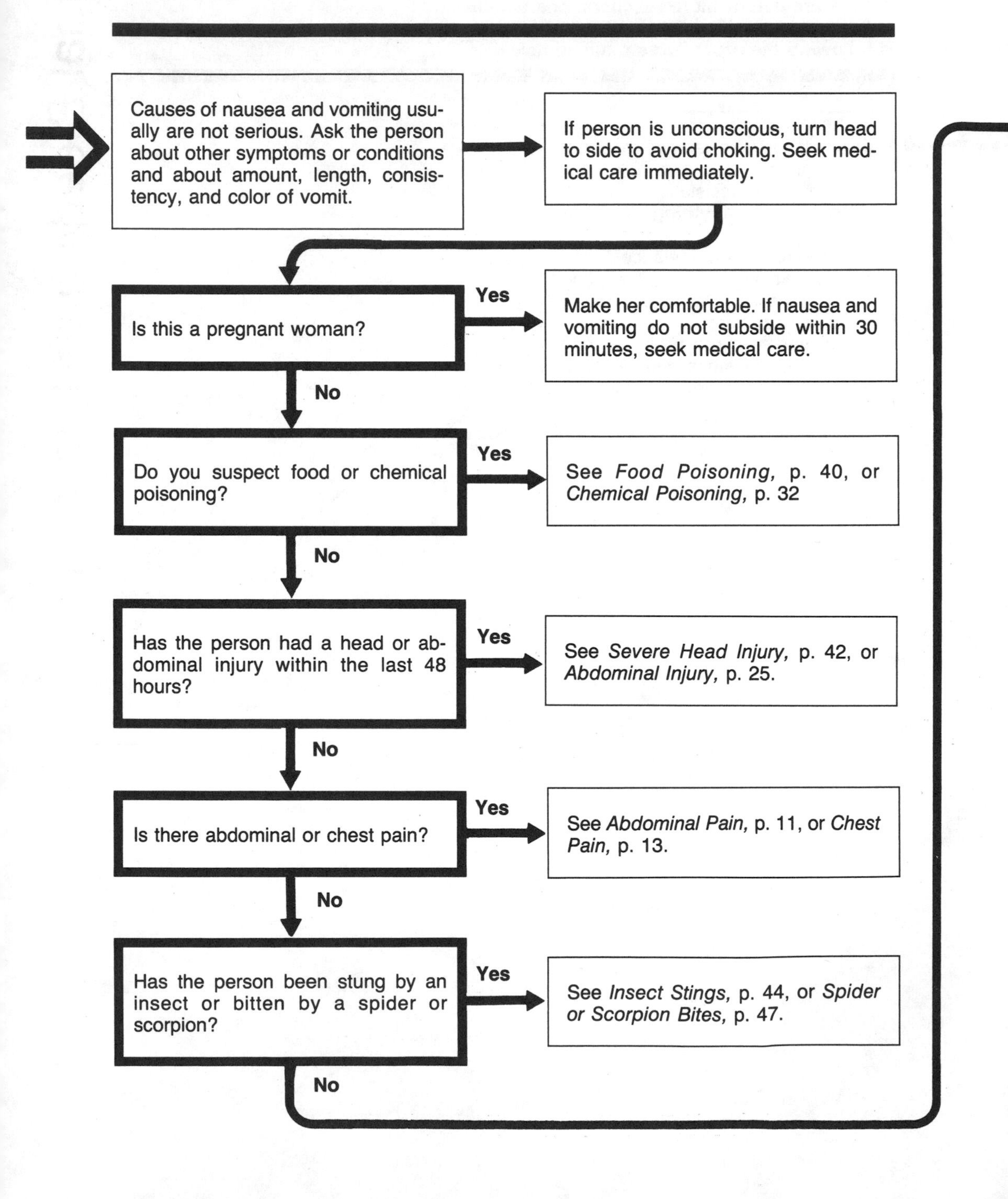

Causes of nausea and vomiting usually are not serious. Ask the person about other symptoms or conditions and about amount, length, consistency, and color of vomit.
If person is unconscious, turn head to side to avoid choking. Seek medical care immediately.
Is this a pregnant woman?
Yes
Make her comfortable. If nausea and vomiting do not subside within 30 minutes, seek medical care.
No
Do you suspect food or chemical poisoning?
Yes
See *Food Poisoning,* p. 40, or *Chemical Poisoning,* p. 32
No
Has the person had a head or abdominal injury within the last 48 hours?
Yes
See *Severe Head Injury,* p. 42, or *Abdominal Injury,* p. 25.
No
Is there abdominal or chest pain?
Yes
See *Abdominal Pain,* p. 11, or *Chest Pain,* p. 13.
No
Has the person been stung by an insect or bitten by a spider or scorpion?
Yes
See *Insect Stings,* p. 44, or *Spider or Scorpion Bites,* p. 47.
No

Calm the person by talking while attending to the problem. Explain what you are doing. Try not to show anxiety; act with confidence. Your calm behavior can help to reassure the sick or injured person.

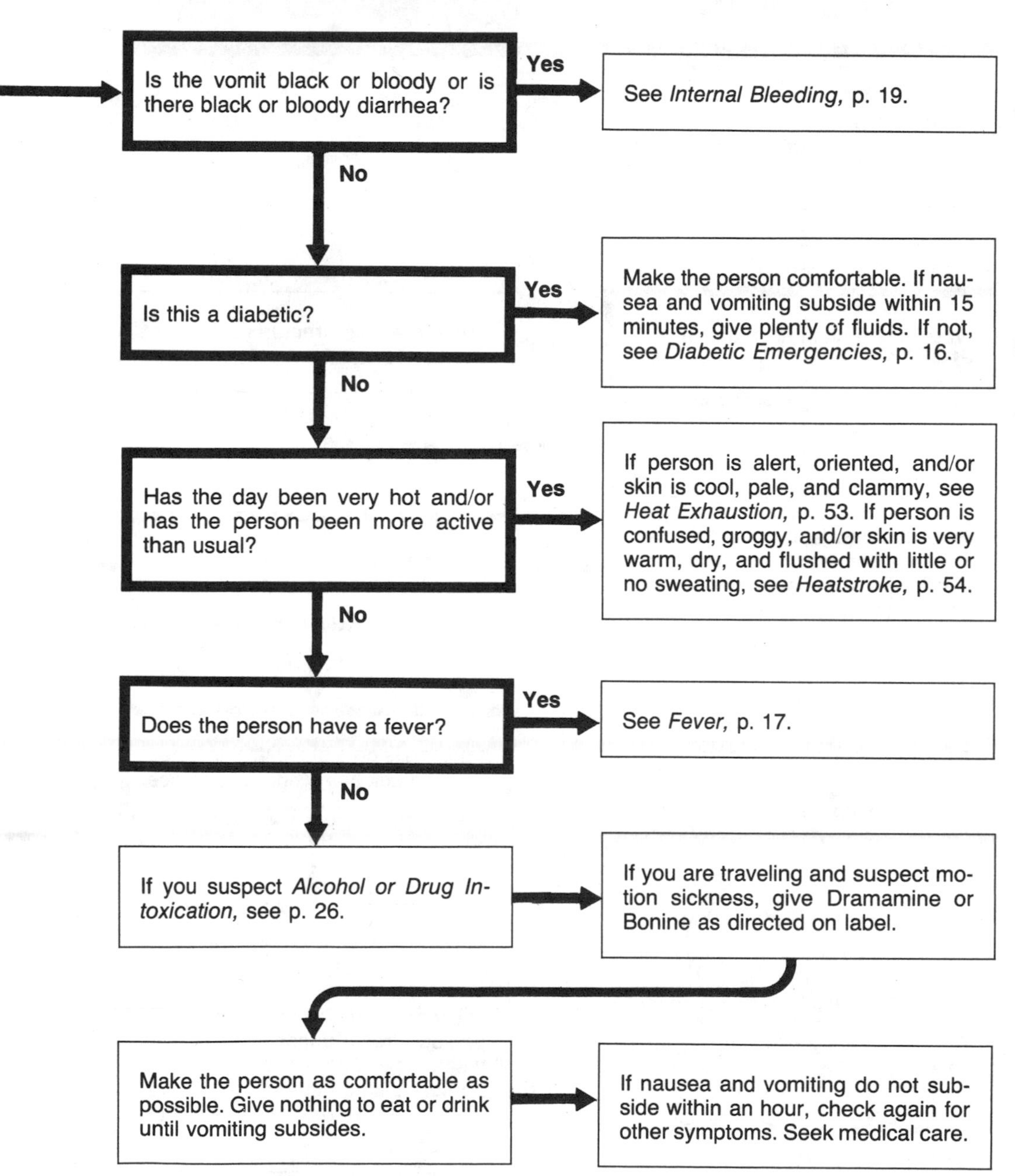
Is the vomit black or bloody or is there black or bloody diarrhea?
Yes
See *Internal Bleeding,* p. 19.
No
Is this a diabetic?
Yes
Make the person comfortable. If nausea and vomiting subside within 15 minutes, give plenty of fluids. If not, see *Diabetic Emergencies,* p. 16.
No
Has the day been very hot and/or has the person been more active than usual?
Yes
If person is alert, oriented, and/or skin is cool, pale, and clammy, see *Heat Exhaustion,* p. 53. If person is confused, groggy, and/or skin is very warm, dry, and flushed with little or no sweating, see *Heatstroke,* p. 54.
No
Does the person have a fever?
Yes
See *Fever,* p. 17.
No
If you suspect *Alcohol or Drug Intoxication,* see p. 26.
If you are traveling and suspect motion sickness, give Dramamine or Bonine as directed on label.
Make the person as comfortable as possible. Give nothing to eat or drink until vomiting subsides.
If nausea and vomiting do not subside within an hour, check again for other symptoms. Seek medical care.

21 Nosebleed

Do not stuff cotton or tissues into the nose.

If person fell or received a head injury, see ***Severe Head Injury*, p. 42.**

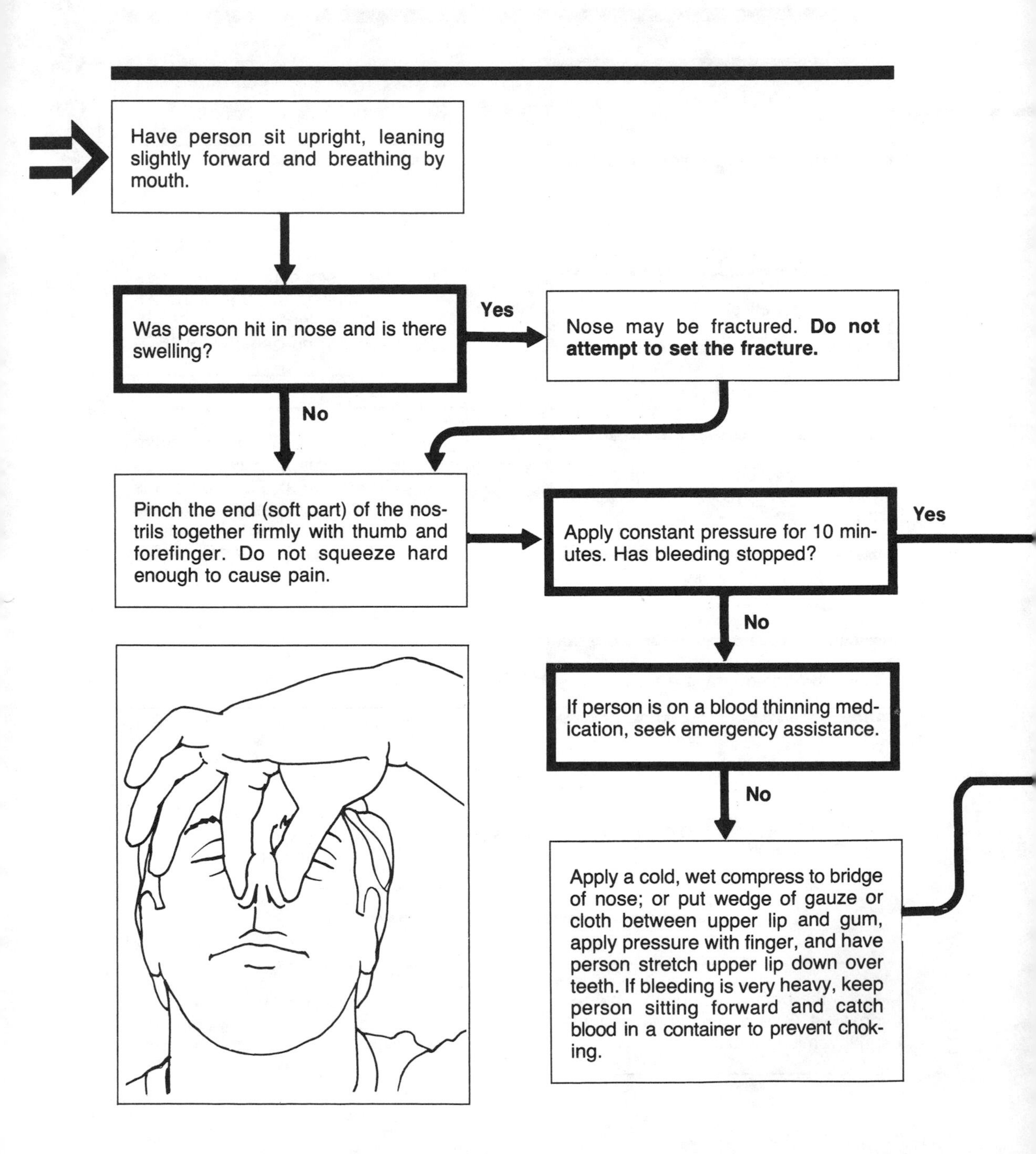

Have person sit upright, leaning slightly forward and breathing by mouth.
Was person hit in nose and is there swelling?
Yes
Nose may be fractured. **Do not attempt to set the fracture.**
No
Pinch the end (soft part) of the nostrils together firmly with thumb and forefinger. Do not squeeze hard enough to cause pain.
Apply constant pressure for 10 minutes. Has bleeding stopped?
Yes
No
If person is on a blood thinning medication, seek emergency assistance.
No
Apply a cold, wet compress to bridge of nose; or put wedge of gauze or cloth between upper lip and gum, apply pressure with finger, and have person stretch upper lip down over teeth. If bleeding is very heavy, keep person sitting forward and catch blood in a container to prevent choking.

Calm the person by talking while attending to the problem. Explain what you are doing. Try not to show anxiety; act with confidence. Your calm behavior can help to reassure the sick or injured person.

If the injury was the result of a vehicular or job-related accident, the person should be examined by a physician for possible additional injuries or complications.

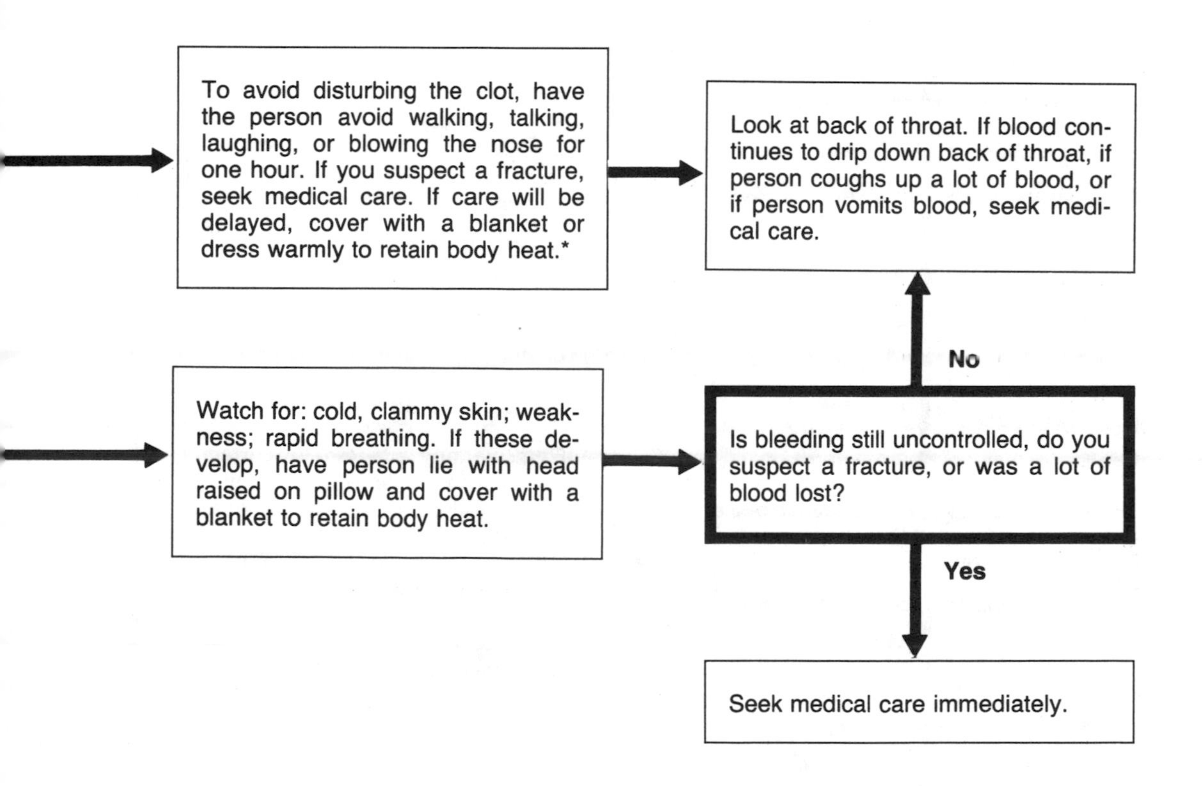
To avoid disturbing the clot, have the person avoid walking, talking, laughing, or blowing the nose for one hour. If you suspect a fracture, seek medical care. If care will be delayed, cover with a blanket or dress warmly to retain body heat.*
Look at back of throat. If blood continues to drip down back of throat, if person coughs up a lot of blood, or if person vomits blood, seek medical care.
No
Watch for: cold, clammy skin; weakness; rapid breathing. If these develop, have person lie with head raised on pillow and cover with a blanket to retain body heat.
Is bleeding still uncontrolled, do you suspect a fracture, or was a lot of blood lost?
Yes
Seek medical care immediately.

*If weather is very warm and person's skin does not feel cool and clammy, covering will not be necessary.

Stroke

Possible Signs & Symptoms: *stiffness or paralysis of facial muscles, extremities, either side of body/breathing or swallowing difficulty/confusion/dizziness/loss of bladder or bowel control/pupils unequal in size/headache/blurred vision/slurred speech or inability to speak/convulsions/unconsciousness/coma*

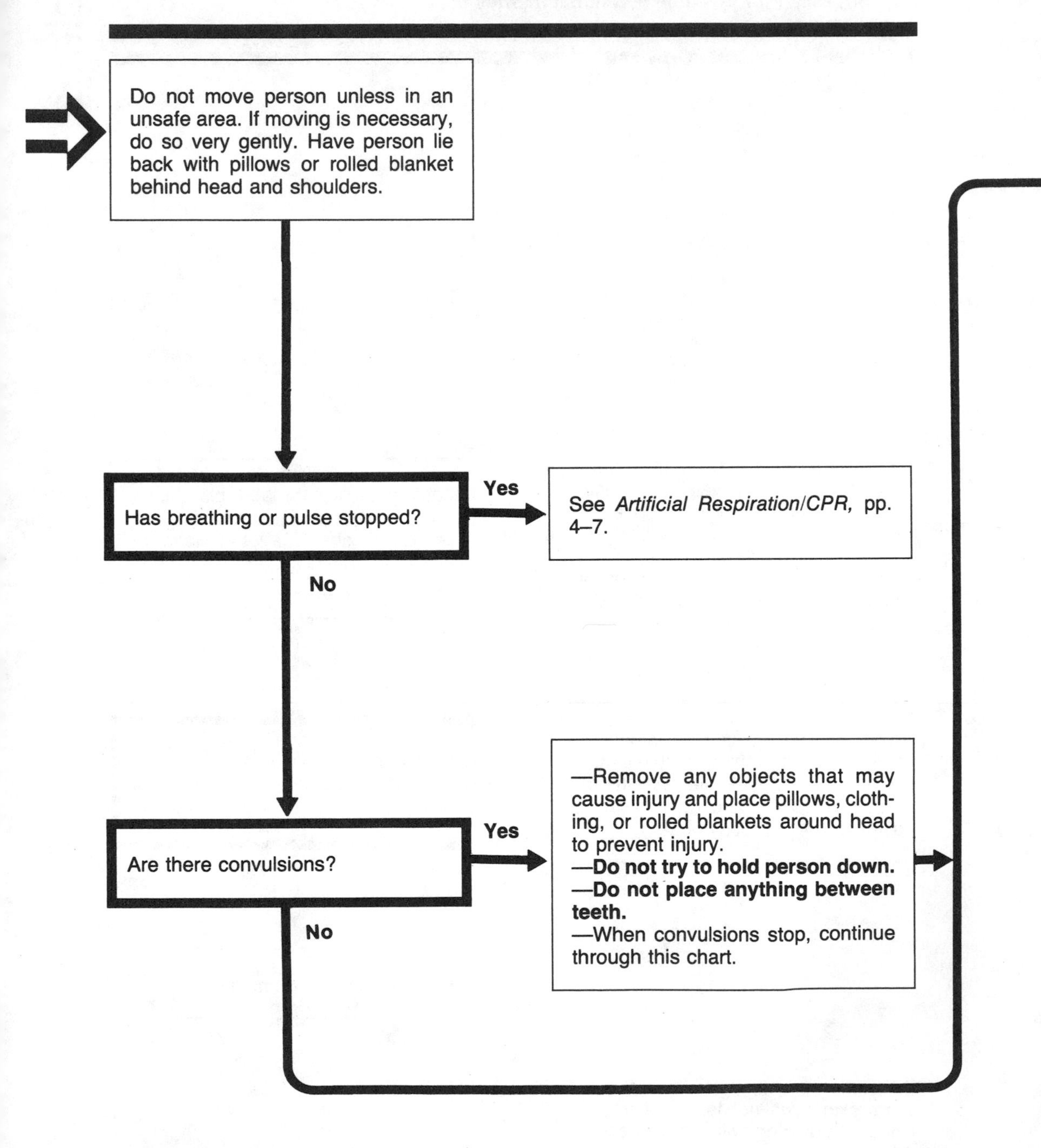

Do not move person unless in an unsafe area. If moving is necessary, do so very gently. Have person lie back with pillows or rolled blanket behind head and shoulders.
Has breathing or pulse stopped?
Yes
See *Artificial Respiration/CPR,* pp. 4–7.
No
Are there convulsions?
Yes
—Remove any objects that may cause injury and place pillows, clothing, or rolled blankets around head to prevent injury.
—Do not try to hold person down.
—Do not place anything between teeth.
—When convulsions stop, continue through this chart.
No

Calm the person by talking while attending to the problem. Explain what you are doing. Try not to show anxiety; act with confidence. Your calm behavior can help to reassure the sick person.

If there are two or more rescuers, one should obtain emergency assistance while the other is following the procedures outlined below.

If the person is unconscious or appears to be choking, turn head to side to allow drainage of secretions. Remove dentures if loose. If necessary, wrap a cloth around your fingers and clear out mouth and throat. **Do not give anything to eat or drink.**

If you do *not* suspect a fracture, gently straighten any twisted or paralyzed limb(s) to maintain proper circulation.

If emergency assistance has not been summoned, obtain help now. While awaiting assistance:
—Continue to check breathing and pulse. If either stops, see *Artificial Respiration/CPR,* pp. 4–7.
—Watch for shock: cold, clammy skin; rapid breathing; weakness. If these develop, cover with blanket or clothing to retain body heat.

23 Toothache or Lost or Broken Tooth

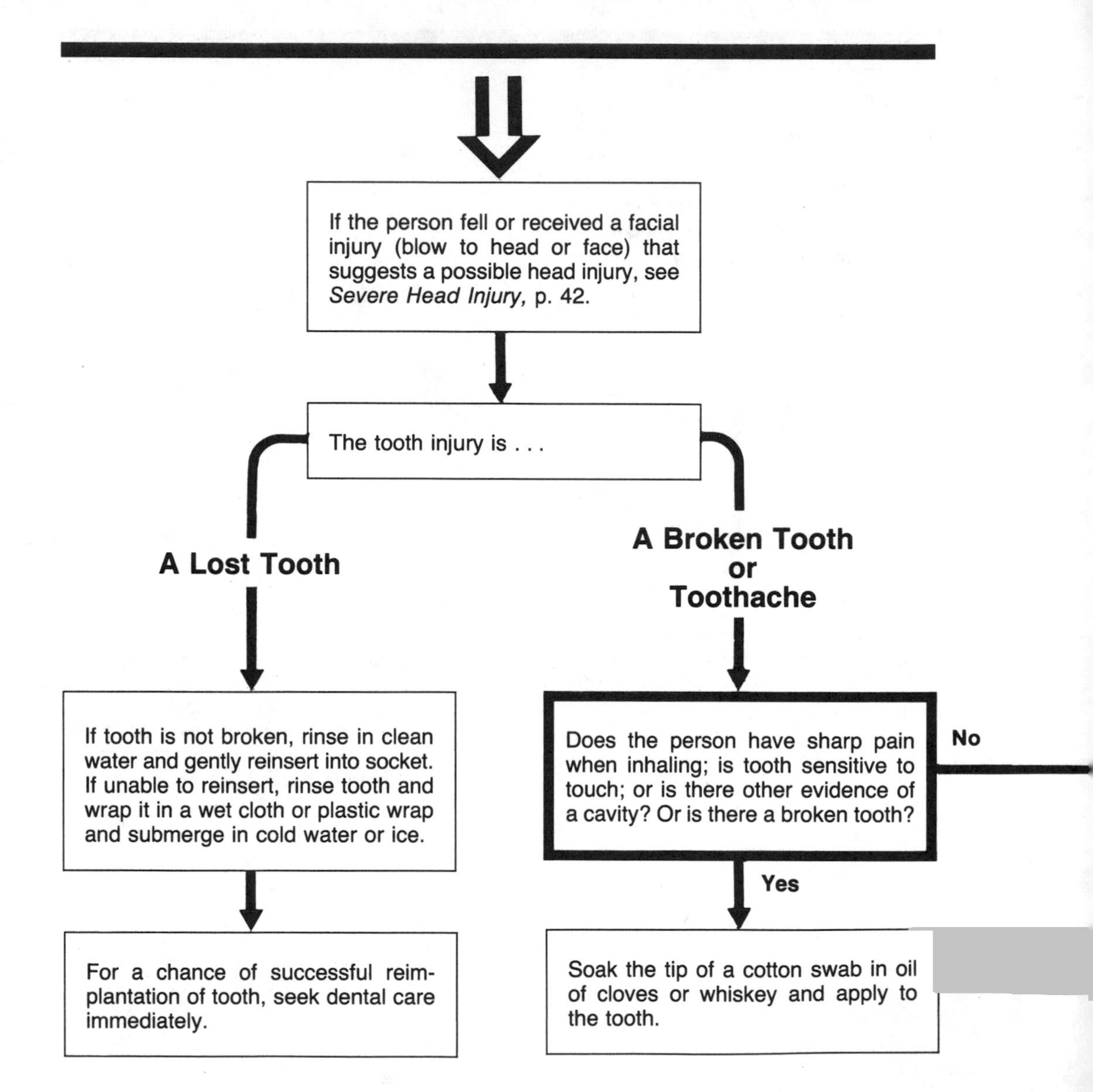

If the person fell or received a facial injury (blow to head or face) that suggests a possible head injury, see *Severe Head Injury*, p. 42.
The tooth injury is . . .
A Lost Tooth
A Broken Tooth or Toothache
If tooth is not broken, rinse in clean water and gently reinsert into socket. If unable to reinsert, rinse tooth and wrap it in a wet cloth or plastic wrap and submerge in cold water or ice.
For a chance of successful reimplantation of tooth, seek dental care immediately.
Does the person have sharp pain when inhaling; is tooth sensitive to touch; or is there other evidence of a cavity? Or is there a broken tooth?
No
Yes
Soak the tip of a cotton swab in oil of cloves or whiskey and apply to the tooth.

Calm the person by talking while attending to the problem. Explain what you are doing. Try not to show anxiety; act with confidence. Your calm behavior can help to reassure the injured person.

If injury was the result of a vehicular or job-related accident, the person should be examined by a physician for possible additional injuries or complications.

Apply warm packs to the side of face to lessen pain.

If dental care is not immediately available, melt or rub between your palms a piece of paraffin or candle; mix in some strands of cotton. When wax mixture begins to cool, apply to the tooth as a temporary filling.

Give aspirin or acetaminophen tablets for pain. Follow label directions.

Have the person rest in a comfortable position. Lying flat may increase pain, so use pillows or rolled blankets behind head and shoulders.

Seek dental care immediately to avoid the possibility of infection developing or progressing.

Unconsciousness

Shout for help even if you think you are alone. If there are two or more rescuers, one should obtain emergency assistance while the other is following the procedures outlined below.

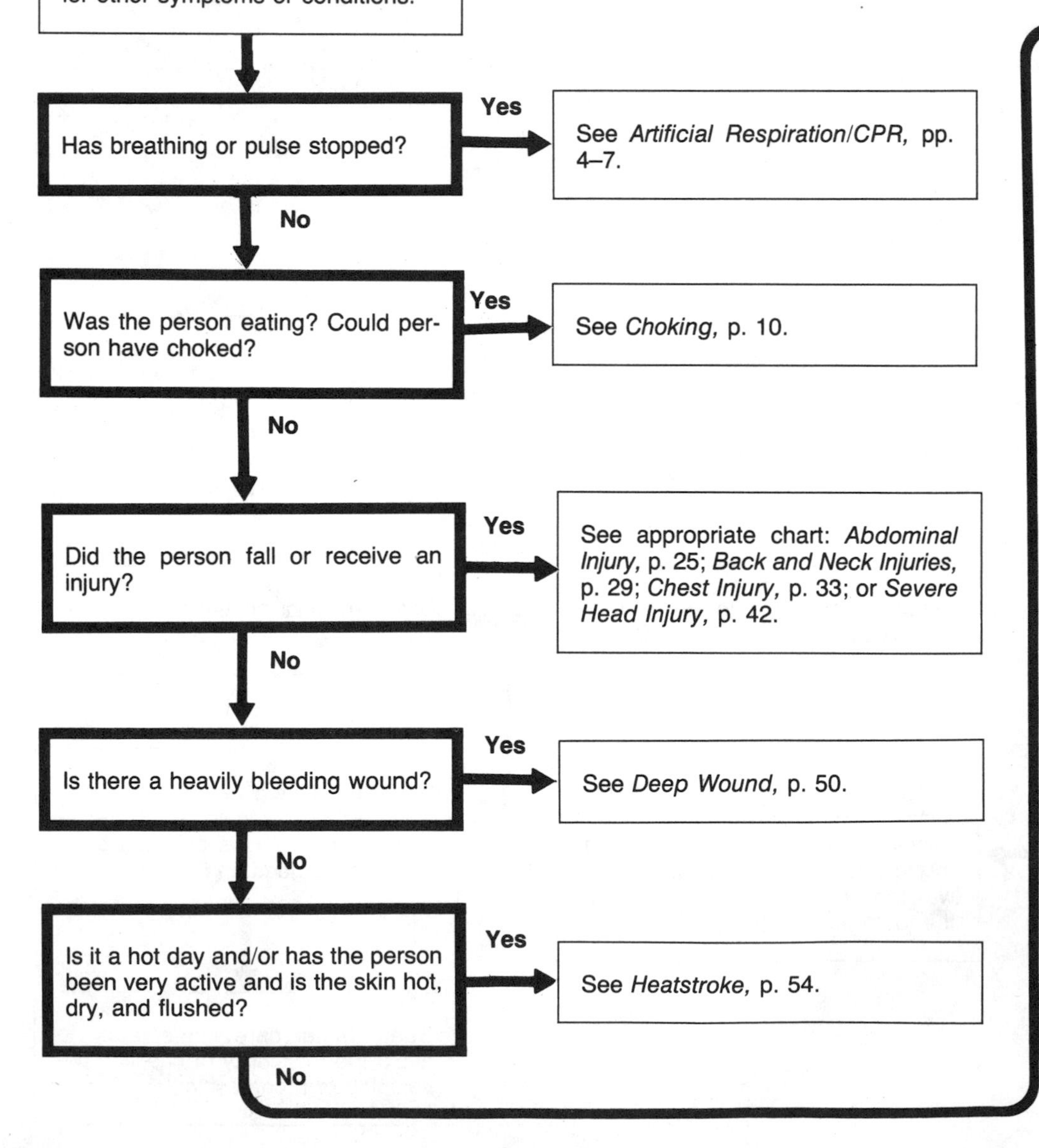
Move the person only if in an unsafe area. If moving is necessary, do so very gently, supporting the neck and back if you suspect injury. (See *Basic Emergency Principles and Transfer Procedures,* p. 2.) Check quickly for other symptoms or conditions.
Has breathing or pulse stopped?
Yes
See *Artificial Respiration/CPR,* pp. 4–7.
No
Was the person eating? Could person have choked?
Yes
See *Choking,* p. 10.
No
Did the person fall or receive an injury?
Yes
See appropriate chart: *Abdominal Injury,* p. 25; *Back and Neck Injuries,* p. 29; *Chest Injury,* p. 33; or *Severe Head Injury,* p. 42.
No
Is there a heavily bleeding wound?
Yes
See *Deep Wound,* p. 50.
No
Is it a hot day and/or has the person been very active and is the skin hot, dry, and flushed?
Yes
See *Heatstroke,* p. 54.
No

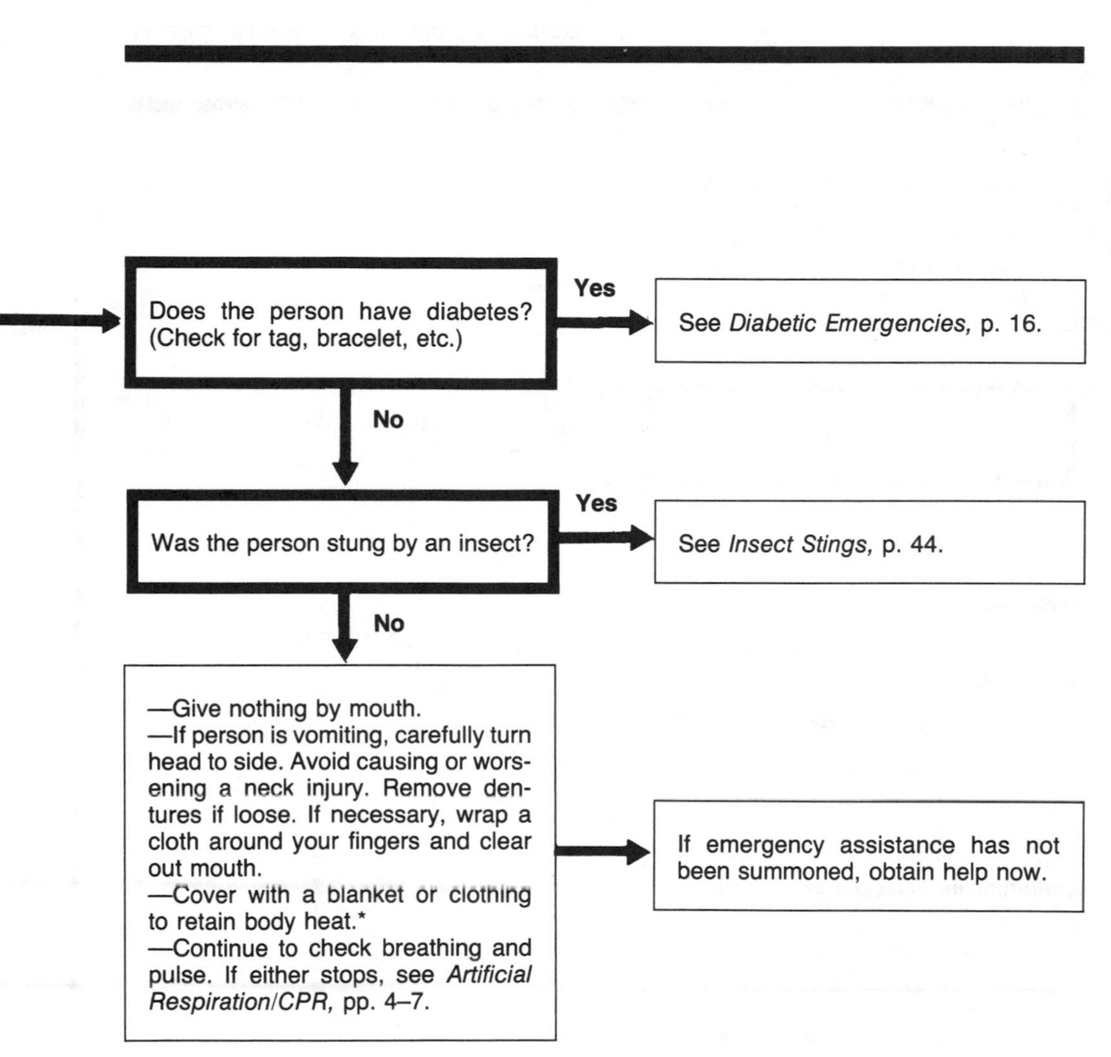
Does the person have diabetes? (Check for tag, bracelet, etc.)
Yes
See *Diabetic Emergencies,* p. 16.
No
Was the person stung by an insect?
Yes
See *Insect Stings,* p. 44.
No
—Give nothing by mouth.
—If person is vomiting, carefully turn head to side. Avoid causing or worsening a neck injury. Remove dentures if loose. If necessary, wrap a cloth around your fingers and clear out mouth.
—Cover with a blanket or clothing to retain body heat.*
—Continue to check breathing and pulse. If either stops, see *Artificial Respiration/CPR,* pp. 4–7.
If emergency assistance has not been summoned, obtain help now.

*If weather is very warm and person's skin does not feel cool and clammy, covering will not be necessary.

25 Abdominal Injury

Signs & Symptoms:
Internal bleeding: swelling/discoloration/ severe pain/cold, clammy skin/restlessness/ thirst/vomiting or coughing blood/blood in urine or feces.
Hernia: pain, swelling, or discoloration in groin or scrotum

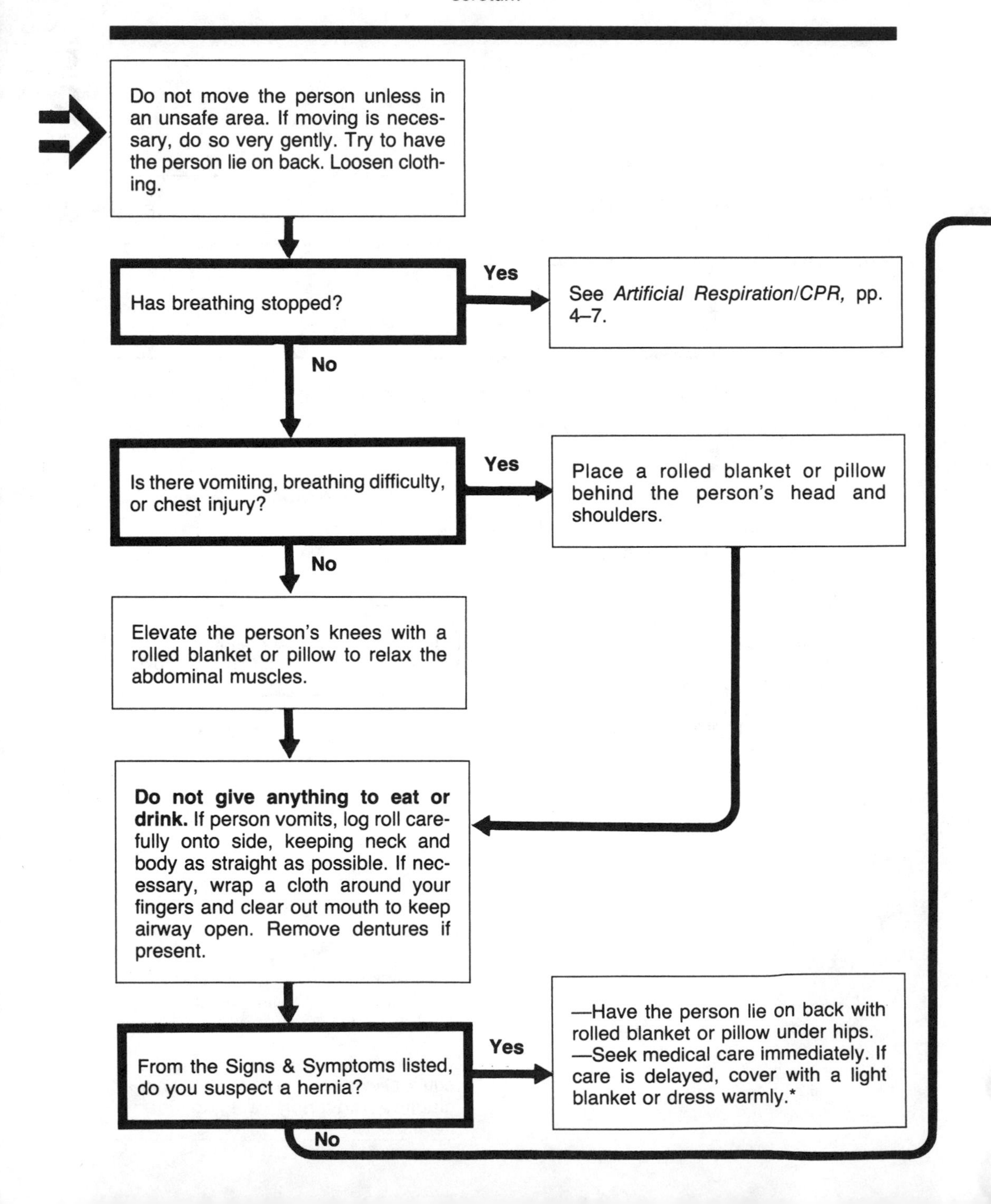

Do not move the person unless in an unsafe area. If moving is necessary, do so very gently. Try to have the person lie on back. Loosen clothing.
Has breathing stopped?
Yes
See Artificial Respiration/CPR, pp. 4–7.
No
Is there vomiting, breathing difficulty, or chest injury?
Yes
Place a rolled blanket or pillow behind the person's head and shoulders.
No
Elevate the person's knees with a rolled blanket or pillow to relax the abdominal muscles.
Do not give anything to eat or drink. If person vomits, log roll carefully onto side, keeping neck and body as straight as possible. If necessary, wrap a cloth around your fingers and clear out mouth to keep airway open. Remove dentures if present.
From the Signs & Symptoms listed, do you suspect a hernia?
Yes
—Have the person lie on back with rolled blanket or pillow under hips.
—Seek medical care immediately. If care is delayed, cover with a light blanket or dress warmly.*
No

Calm the person by talking while attending to the problem. Explain what you are doing. Try not to show anxiety; act with confidence. Your calm behavior can help to reassure the injured person. **If there was a severe blow to the head or a fall, or if person is unconscious, assume neck injury and do not move.**

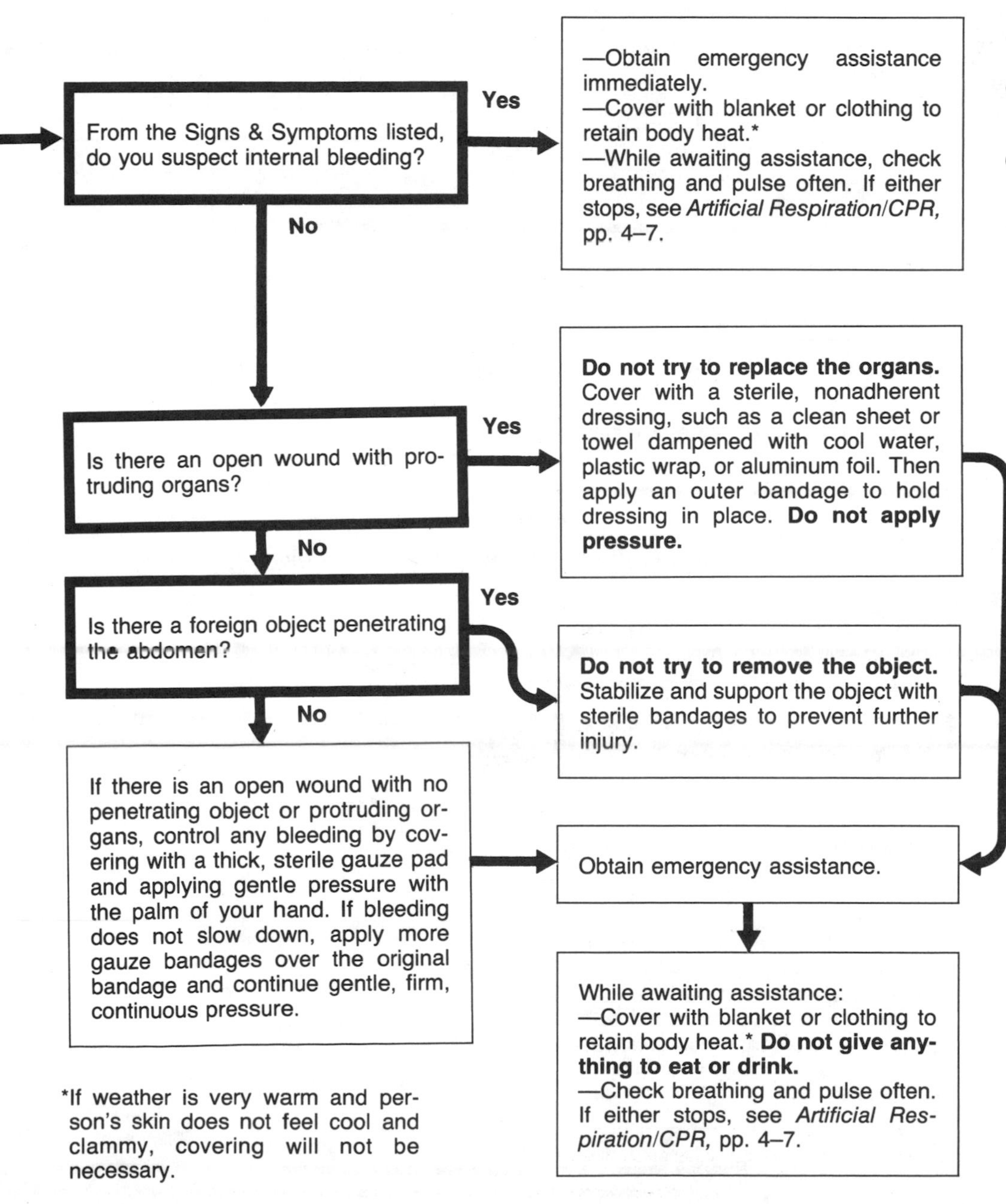
From the Signs & Symptoms listed, do you suspect internal bleeding?
Yes
—Obtain emergency assistance immediately.
—Cover with blanket or clothing to retain body heat.*
—While awaiting assistance, check breathing and pulse often. If either stops, see Artificial Respiration/CPR, pp. 4–7.
No
Is there an open wound with protruding organs?
Yes
Do not try to replace the organs. Cover with a sterile, nonadherent dressing, such as a clean sheet or towel dampened with cool water, plastic wrap, or aluminum foil. Then apply an outer bandage to hold dressing in place. Do not apply pressure.
No
Is there a foreign object penetrating the abdomen?
Yes
Do not try to remove the object. Stabilize and support the object with sterile bandages to prevent further injury.
No
If there is an open wound with no penetrating object or protruding organs, control any bleeding by covering with a thick, sterile gauze pad and applying gentle pressure with the palm of your hand. If bleeding does not slow down, apply more gauze bandages over the original bandage and continue gentle, firm, continuous pressure.
Obtain emergency assistance.
While awaiting assistance:
—Cover with blanket or clothing to retain body heat.* Do not give anything to eat or drink.
—Check breathing and pulse often. If either stops, see Artificial Respiration/CPR, pp. 4–7.

*If weather is very warm and person's skin does not feel cool and clammy, covering will not be necessary.

Alcohol or Drug Intoxication

Possible Signs & Symptoms: *restlessness/ confusion/slurred speech/flushed skin/hallucinations/pinpoint or dilated pupils/muscular twitching/tremors/nausea and vomiting/ drowsiness/shallow breathing/cold sweat/ dizziness/irritability/fear/depression/violent or aggressive behavior/convulsions/unconsciousness. Symptoms will vary with different drugs.*
For Allergic Reaction, see p. 27.

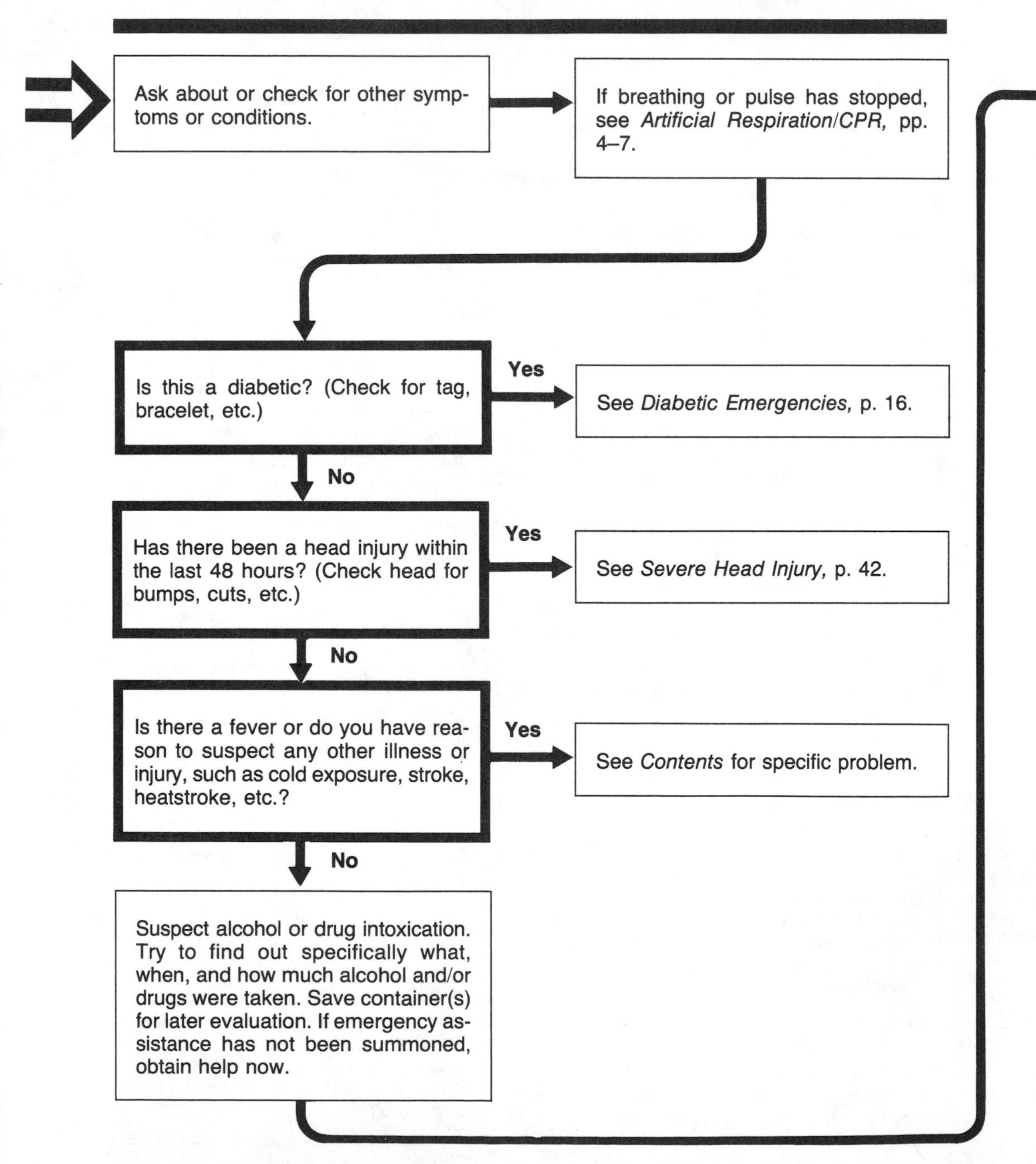

Ask about or check for other symptoms or conditions.
If breathing or pulse has stopped, see *Artificial Respiration/CPR,* pp. 4–7.
Is this a diabetic? (Check for tag, bracelet, etc.)
Yes
See *Diabetic Emergencies,* p. 16.
No
Has there been a head injury within the last 48 hours? (Check head for bumps, cuts, etc.)
Yes
See *Severe Head Injury,* p. 42.
No
Is there a fever or do you have reason to suspect any other illness or injury, such as cold exposure, stroke, heatstroke, etc.?
Yes
See *Contents* for specific problem.
No
Suspect alcohol or drug intoxication. Try to find out specifically what, when, and how much alcohol and/or drugs were taken. Save container(s) for later evaluation. If emergency assistance has not been summoned, obtain help now.

Calm the person by talking while attending to the problem. Explain what you are doing. Try not to show anxiety; act with confidence. Your calm behavior can help to reassure the sick person.

If there are two or more rescuers, one should obtain emergency assistance while the other is following the procedures outlined below.

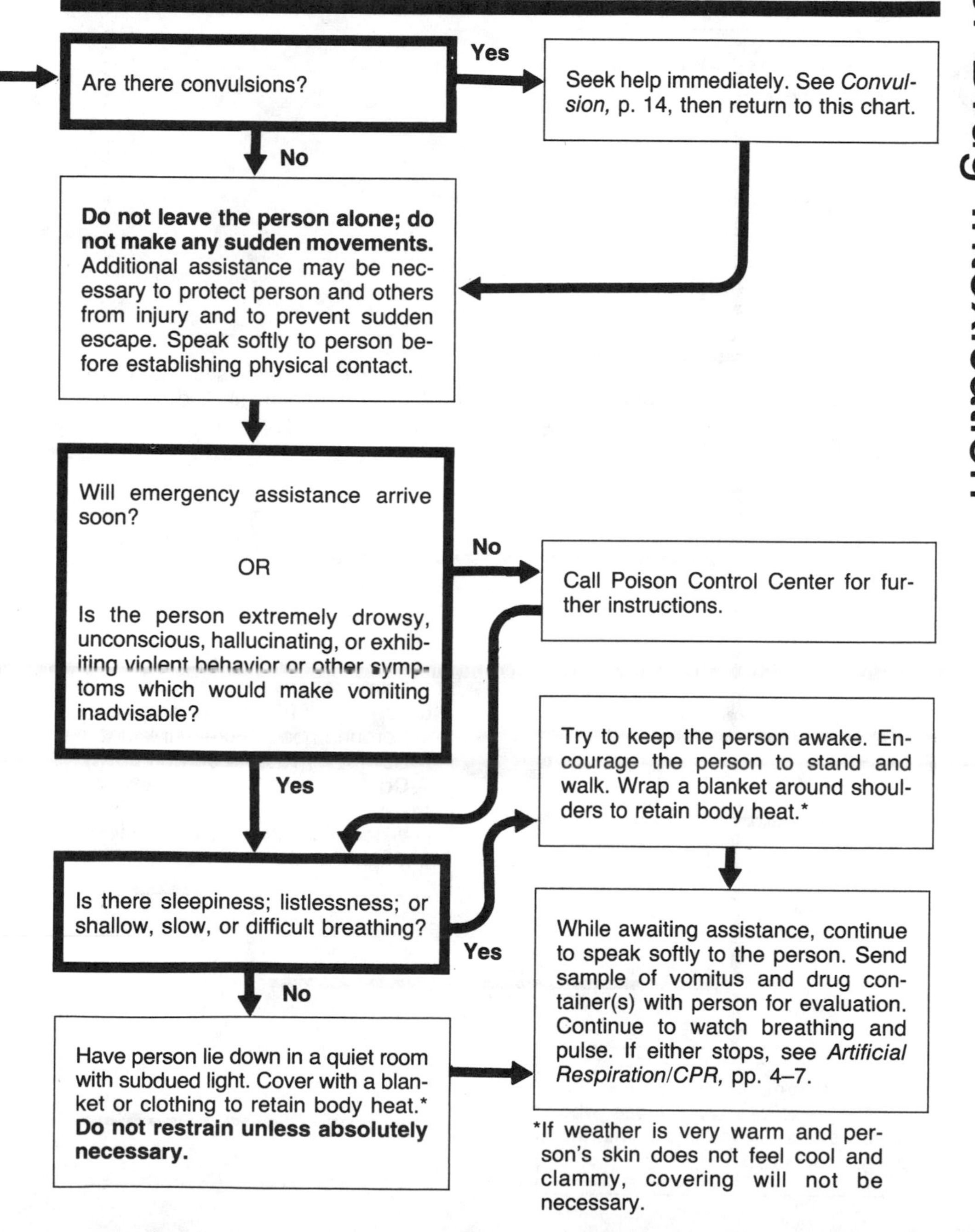

Are there convulsions?
Yes
Seek help immediately. See *Convulsion,* p. 14, then return to this chart.
No
Do not leave the person alone; do not make any sudden movements. Additional assistance may be necessary to protect person and others from injury and to prevent sudden escape. Speak softly to person before establishing physical contact.
Will emergency assistance arrive soon?
OR
Is the person extremely drowsy, unconscious, hallucinating, or exhibiting violent behavior or other symptoms which would make vomiting inadvisable?
No
Call Poison Control Center for further instructions.
Yes
Is there sleepiness; listlessness; or shallow, slow, or difficult breathing?
Yes
Try to keep the person awake. Encourage the person to stand and walk. Wrap a blanket around shoulders to retain body heat.*
No
Have person lie down in a quiet room with subdued light. Cover with a blanket or clothing to retain body heat.* **Do not restrain unless absolutely necessary.**
While awaiting assistance, continue to speak softly to the person. Send sample of vomitus and drug container(s) with person for evaluation. Continue to watch breathing and pulse. If either stops, see *Artificial Respiration/CPR,* pp. 4–7.

*If weather is very warm and person's skin does not feel cool and clammy, covering will not be necessary.

27 Allergic Reaction

For drug intoxication with no allergic reaction, see *Alcohol or Drug Intoxication,* p. 26.

Possible Signs & Symptoms: *itching, flushing, or burning, especially near face or chest/hives/edema, particularly of face, neck, tongue, and lips/tightness or pain in chest or throat/coughing or wheezing/breathing difficulty/pale skin/dizziness/convulsions/unconsciousness/coma*

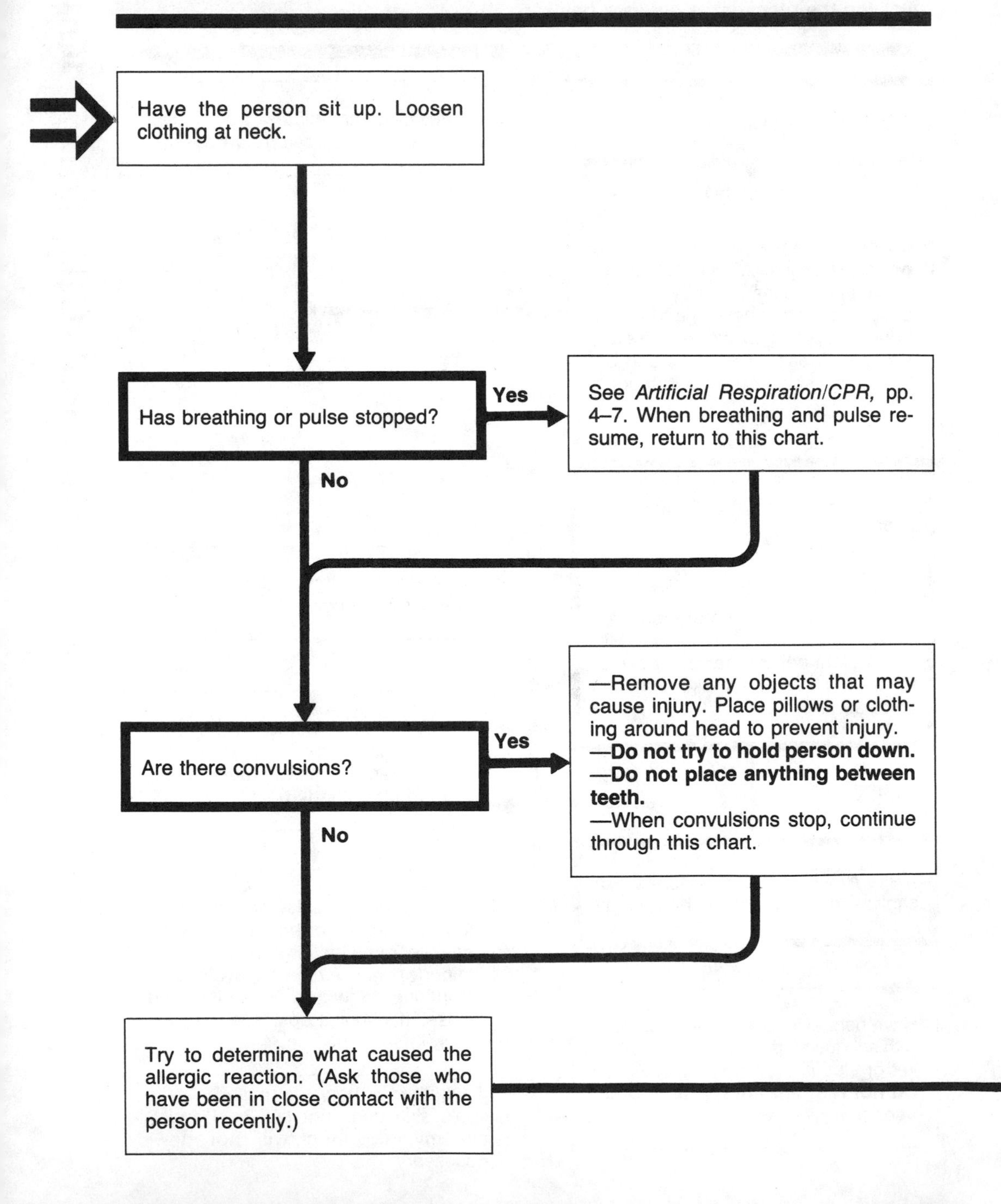
Have the person sit up. Loosen clothing at neck.
Has breathing or pulse stopped?
Yes
See *Artificial Respiration/CPR,* pp. 4–7. When breathing and pulse resume, return to this chart.
No
Are there convulsions?
Yes
—Remove any objects that may cause injury. Place pillows or clothing around head to prevent injury.
—**Do not try to hold person down.**
—**Do not place anything between teeth.**
—When convulsions stop, continue through this chart.
No
Try to determine what caused the allergic reaction. (Ask those who have been in close contact with the person recently.)

Calm the person by talking while attending to the problem. Explain what you are doing. Try not to show anxiety; act with confidence. Your calm behavior can help to reassure the sick person.

If there are two or more rescuers, one should obtain emergency assistance while the other is following the procedures outlined below.

Is this a severe insect sting or drug injection reaction with extensive swelling, loss of consciousness, or difficulty breathing?

Yes

—If an insect bite kit is available, follow instructions, injecting epinephrine first. **Do not inject into limb with original injection site.**
—If kit is unavailable, assistance is delayed, and the person is conscious but having breathing difficulty, give antihistamine (Benadryl) or use epinephrine inhaler (Primatene Mist, etc.), following label directions.
—**Do not give anything by mouth if unconscious.**
—Apply ice wrapped in towel or cold compresses to the site.

If the sting or injection site was on an arm or leg, tie a cloth strip above the site. Band should be snug, but you should still be able to feel the pulse. Keep the sting or injection site below heart level.

If emergency assistance has not been summoned, obtain help now.

While awaiting assistance:
—Loosen the band for 15 seconds every 10–15 minutes.
—**Do not give anything to eat or drink.**
—Continue to check breathing and pulse. If either stops, see *Artificial Respiration/CPR,* pp. 4–7.

No

If assistance will be delayed and there is breathing difficulty caused by swallowing food or drugs, give antihistamine (Benadryl) or use epinephrine inhaler (Primatene Mist, etc.), following label directions. **Do not give anything by mouth if unconscious.**

If emergency assistance has not been summoned, obtain help now.

While awaiting assistance:
—**Do not give anything to eat or drink.**
—Continue to check breathing and pulse. If either stops, see *Artificial Respiration/CPR,* pp. 4–7.

Animal & Human Bites

If there are two or more rescuers, one should attend to the person, while the other tries to trap animal to check later for rabies. **Be careful not to get bitten.** If capturing the animal is not possible, note behavior for later evaluation. (All animal and human bites must be reported to local police and/or health officer.)

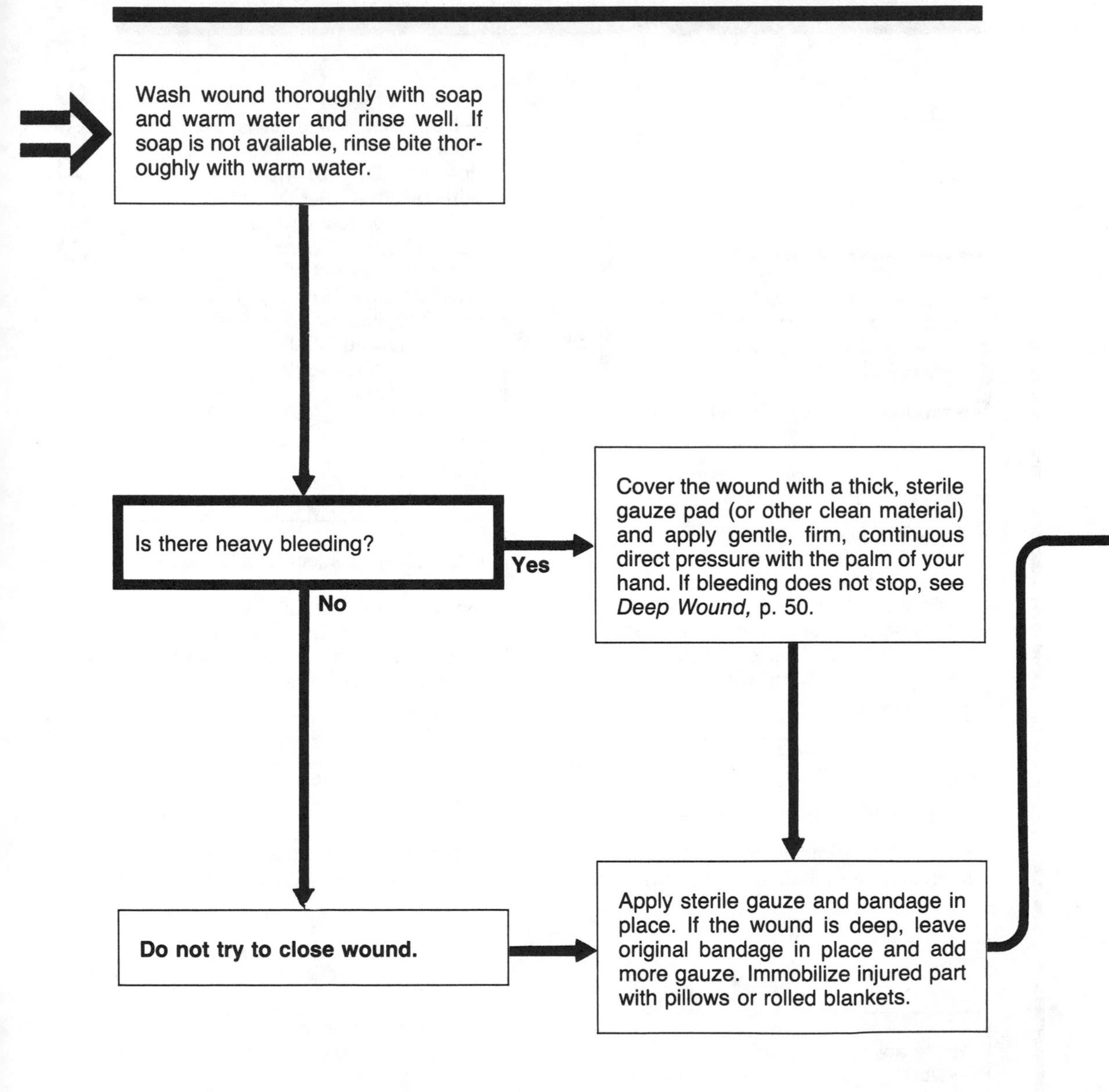

Wash wound thoroughly with soap and warm water and rinse well. If soap is not available, rinse bite thoroughly with warm water.
Is there heavy bleeding?
Yes
No
Cover the wound with a thick, sterile gauze pad (or other clean material) and apply gentle, firm, continuous direct pressure with the palm of your hand. If bleeding does not stop, see *Deep Wound,* p. 50.
Do not try to close wound.
Apply sterile gauze and bandage in place. If the wound is deep, leave original bandage in place and add more gauze. Immobilize injured part with pillows or rolled blankets.

Calm the person by talking while attending to the problem. Explain what you are doing. Try not to show anxiety; act with confidence. Your calm behavior can help to reassure the injured person.

If the wounds are severe, check for breathing and pulse. If either stops, see *Artificial Respiration/CPR*,. pp. 4–7.

Watch for: cold, clammy skin; weakness; rapid breathing. If these develop, cover with a blanket or clothing to retain body heat. If no heart problems or head injuries are present, elevate the legs on a pillow or rolled blanket.

Make person comfortable. Seek medical care. Person may require tetanus immunization and possibly rabies vaccination.

29 Back & Neck Injuries

Signs & Symptoms: *severe pain and tenderness at site of injury/possible deformity of injured area/possible paralysis of one or more limbs/pain on movement*

Do not move someone with severe back or neck injuries unless absolutely necessary.

With any severe fall or other trauma injuring the back, assume fractures of both neck and back. If person is unconscious or groggy from a fall or blow to the head, assume neck fracture.

Secure the neck very carefully with a collar (use rolled towel). Be sure to keep the head straight; do not raise or lower chin or turn head.

→

If breathing or pulse has stopped, gently log roll person onto back, keeping neck and back as straight as possible. See *Artificial Respiration/CPR,* pp. 4–7.

↓

Is the person lying in a safe area?

Yes → Leave in present position. Immobilize by placing pillows or rolled blankets around entire body. Cover with a blanket to retain body heat.* Obtain emergency assistance. Check breathing and pulse often. If either stops, see *Artificial Respiration/CPR,* pp. 4–7.

No ↓

Are there two or more rescuers?
AND
Is a spineboard or makeshift board (mattress board, ironing board, door, leaf from a table, etc.) available?

No →

Yes →

—Place a spineboard or makeshift board beside the person.
—*Rescuers:* Position yourselves as shown below, then grasp with both hands the seams on the side of person's clothing nearest board.
—*Rescuer at the head:* Direct the turning of the body simultaneously and slowly, rolling the person toward the rescuers, keeping the body and head straight.

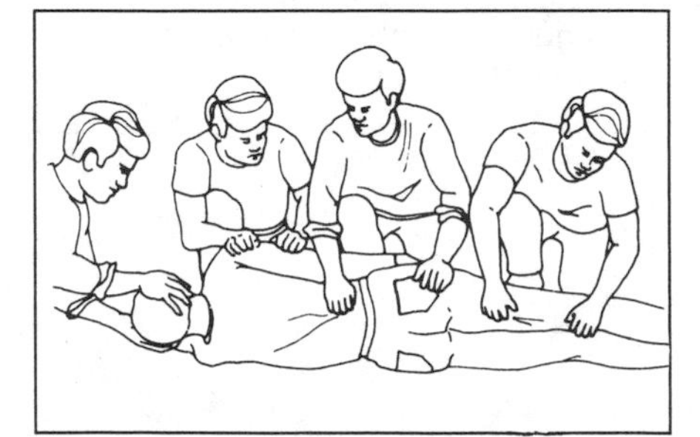

→

—The middle rescuer slides the board underneath the person with one arm, while the others hold the person in place. Then roll the person back simultaneously and slowly, keeping the body and head straight.
—Immobilize the person's head with pillows, towels, etc., without lifting or moving the head.
—Secure the person to the board with belts, ties, straps, rope, etc.
—Then lift the board slowly and simultaneously and walk carefully to safety.
—Obtain emergency assistance.
—While waiting for help, make person comfortable and cover with a blanket to retain body heat.* Check breathing and pulse often. If either stops, see *Artificial Respiration/CPR,* pp. 4–7.

Calm the person by talking while attending to the problem. Explain what you are doing. Try not to show anxiety; act with confidence. Your calm behavior can help to reassure the injured person.

Place your hands under the armpits and cradle the neck and head with your forearms. Gently pull to safety, keeping body straight. Cover with a blanket or clothing to retain body heat.*

Immobilize by placing pillows or rolled blankets around entire body. Obtain emergency assistance. While awaiting assistance, watch breathing and pulse. If either stops, see *Artificial Respiration/CPR,* pp. 4–7.

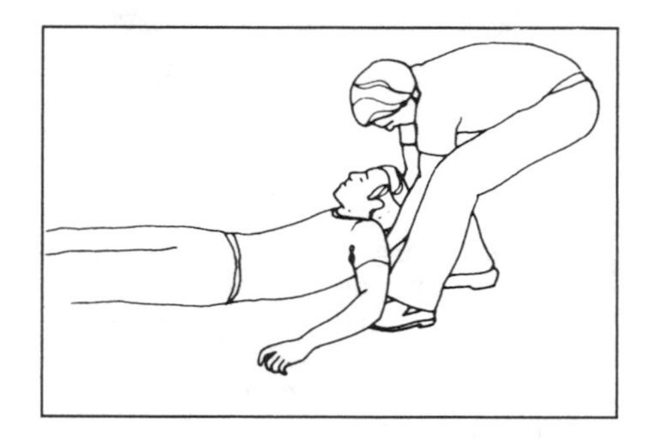

*If weather is very warm and person's skin does not feel cool and clammy, covering will not be necessary.

Bruise

Signs & Symptoms: *pain and tenderness at site of injury/black and blue appearance of skin (may be delayed, with redness appearing first)*

For severe bruise on head, see *Severe Head Injury,* p. 42.

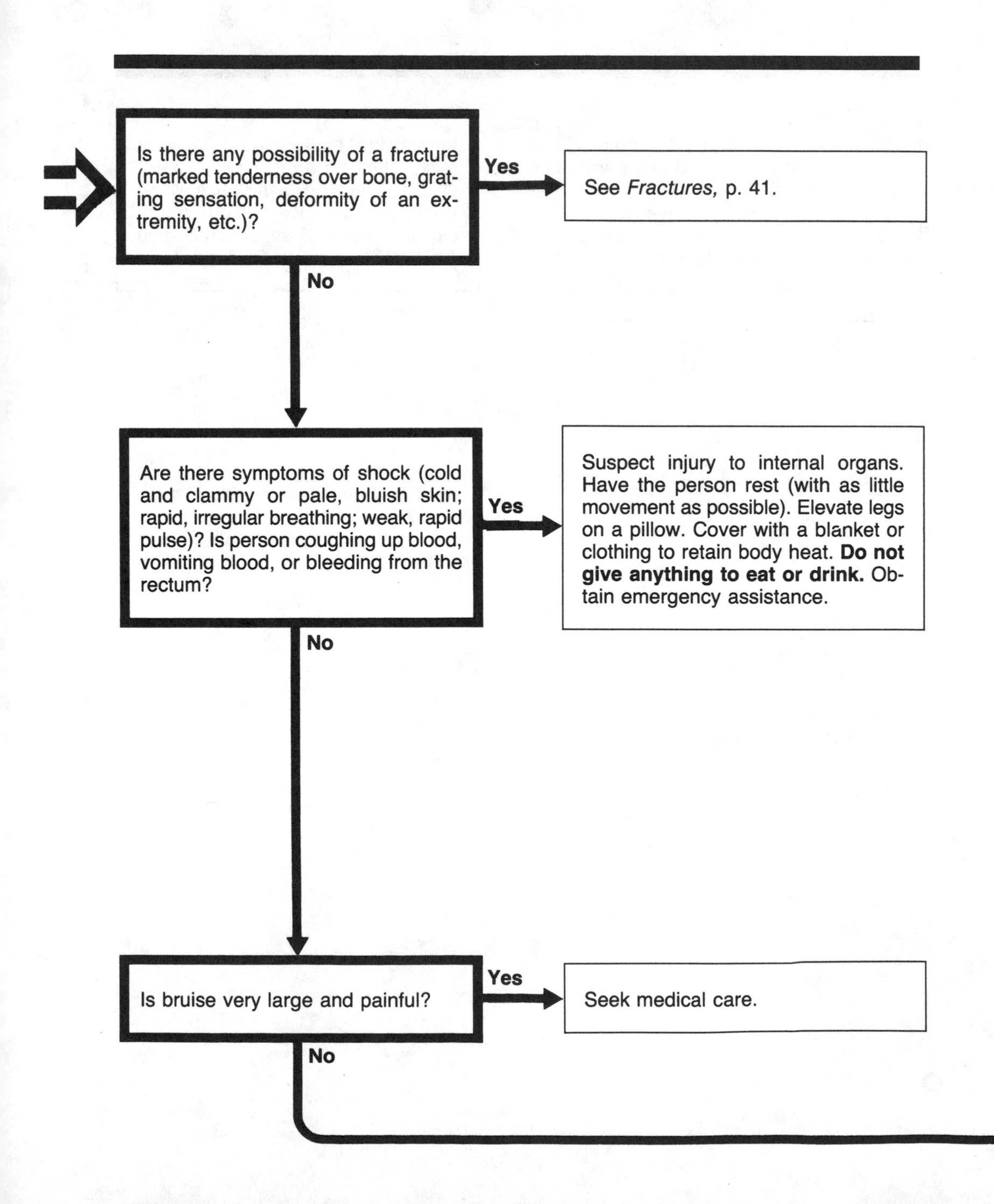

Is there any possibility of a fracture (marked tenderness over bone, grating sensation, deformity of an extremity, etc.)?
Yes
See *Fractures,* p. 41.
No
Are there symptoms of shock (cold and clammy or pale, bluish skin; rapid, irregular breathing; weak, rapid pulse)? Is person coughing up blood, vomiting blood, or bleeding from the rectum?
Yes
Suspect injury to internal organs. Have the person rest (with as little movement as possible). Elevate legs on a pillow. Cover with a blanket or clothing to retain body heat. **Do not give anything to eat or drink.** Obtain emergency assistance.
No
Is bruise very large and painful?
Yes
Seek medical care.
No

Calm the person by talking while attending to the problem. Explain what you are doing. Try not to show anxiety; act with confidence. Your calm behavior can help to reassure the injured person.

If injury was the result of a vehicular or job-related accident, the person should be examined by a physician for possible additional injuries or complications.

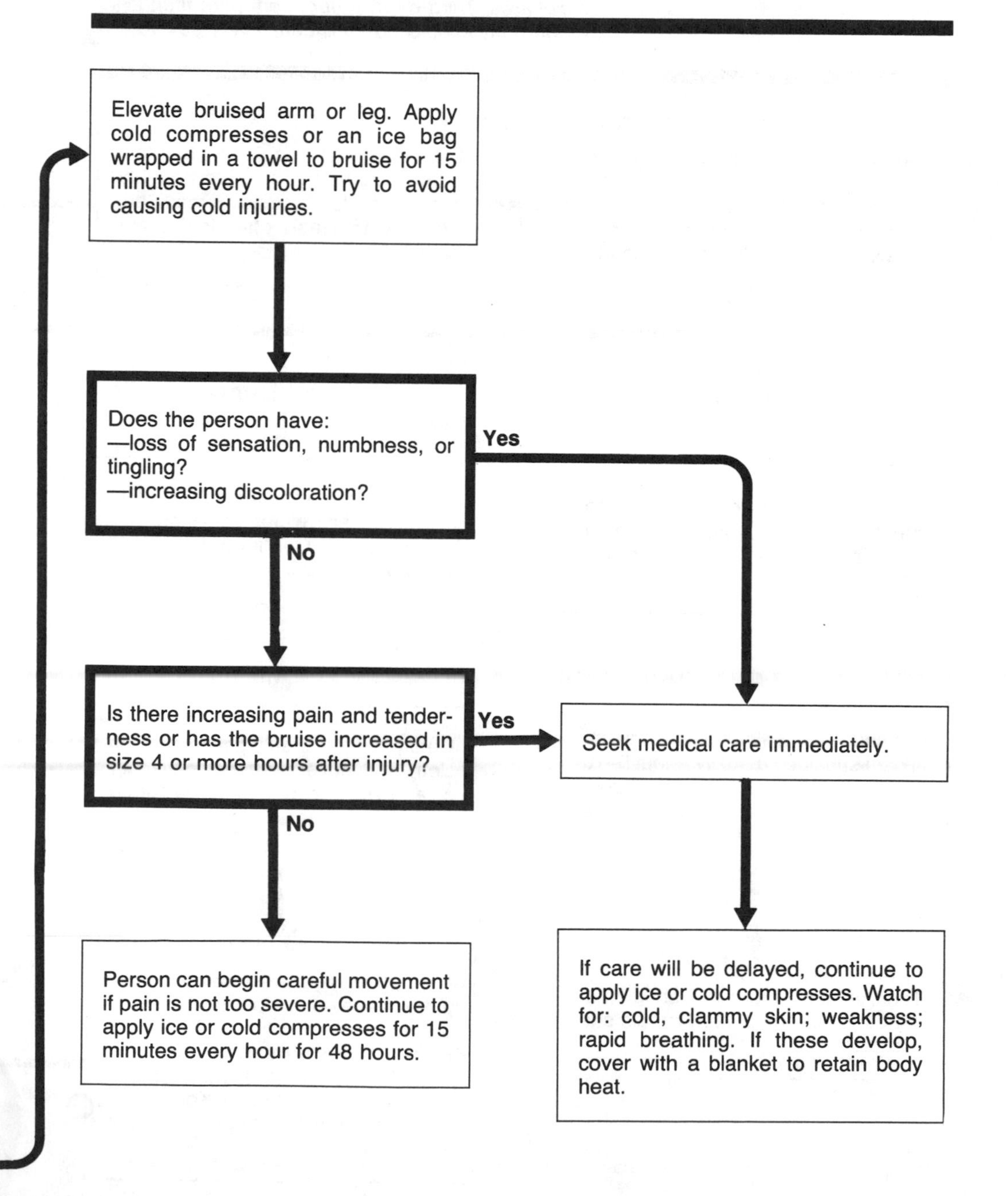

Elevate bruised arm or leg. Apply cold compresses or an ice bag wrapped in a towel to bruise for 15 minutes every hour. Try to avoid causing cold injuries.
Does the person have:
—loss of sensation, numbness, or tingling?
—increasing discoloration?
Yes
No
Is there increasing pain and tenderness or has the bruise increased in size 4 or more hours after injury?
Yes
No
Seek medical care immediately.
Person can begin careful movement if pain is not too severe. Continue to apply ice or cold compresses for 15 minutes every hour for 48 hours.
If care will be delayed, continue to apply ice or cold compresses. Watch for: cold, clammy skin; weakness; rapid breathing. If these develop, cover with a blanket to retain body heat.

31 Burns

(Including Lightning, Electric Shock, Chemical Burns, and Sunburn)

First Degree: *redness of skin/pain, perhaps with mild swelling.*
Second Degree: *deep reddening of skin/glossy appearance from leaking fluid (plasma)/possible loss of some skin/blisters. Second degree burns involving over 10% of the body should be considered severe.*
Third Degree: *loss of all skin layers/possible charring of skin edges/involving more than a very small area. Third degree burns on more than 2% of the body should be considered very severe.*

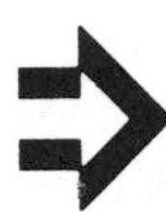

If person is unconscious, check breathing and pulse. If either has stopped, see *Artificial Respiration/CPR,* pp. 4–7. When breathing and/or pulse resume, return to this chart.

If person has received chemical burns, flush the area thoroughly with water for at least 5 minutes. **Be sure to wash chemical away completely.**

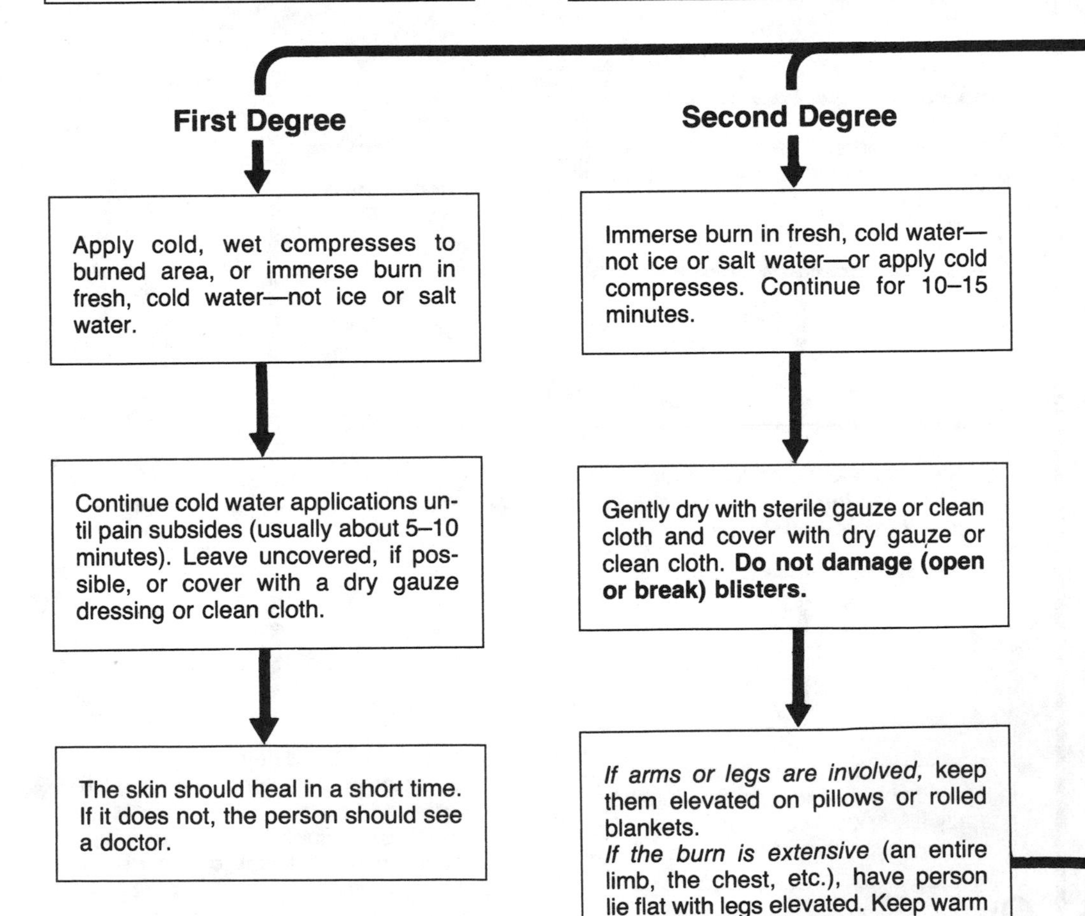
First Degree
Apply cold, wet compresses to burned area, or immerse burn in fresh, cold water—not ice or salt water.
Continue cold water applications until pain subsides (usually about 5–10 minutes). Leave uncovered, if possible, or cover with a dry gauze dressing or clean cloth.
The skin should heal in a short time. If it does not, the person should see a doctor.
Second Degree
Immerse burn in fresh, cold water—not ice or salt water—or apply cold compresses. Continue for 10–15 minutes.
Gently dry with sterile gauze or clean cloth and cover with dry gauze or clean cloth. Do not damage (open or break) blisters.
If arms or legs are involved, keep them elevated on pillows or rolled blankets.
If the burn is extensive (an entire limb, the chest, etc.), have person lie flat with legs elevated. Keep warm by covering with a clean sheet and a blanket.*

In cases of electric shock, if person is still touching electrical source, do not touch either the person or the source. First, turn off master electrical switch or pull appliance plug. If caused by fallen electrical wire, do not try to move the wire away. Instead, obtain emergency assistance (i.e., police, fire departments, etc.)

Calm the person by talking while attending to the problem. Explain what you are doing. Try not to show anxiety; act with confidence. Your calm behavior can help to reassure the injured person.

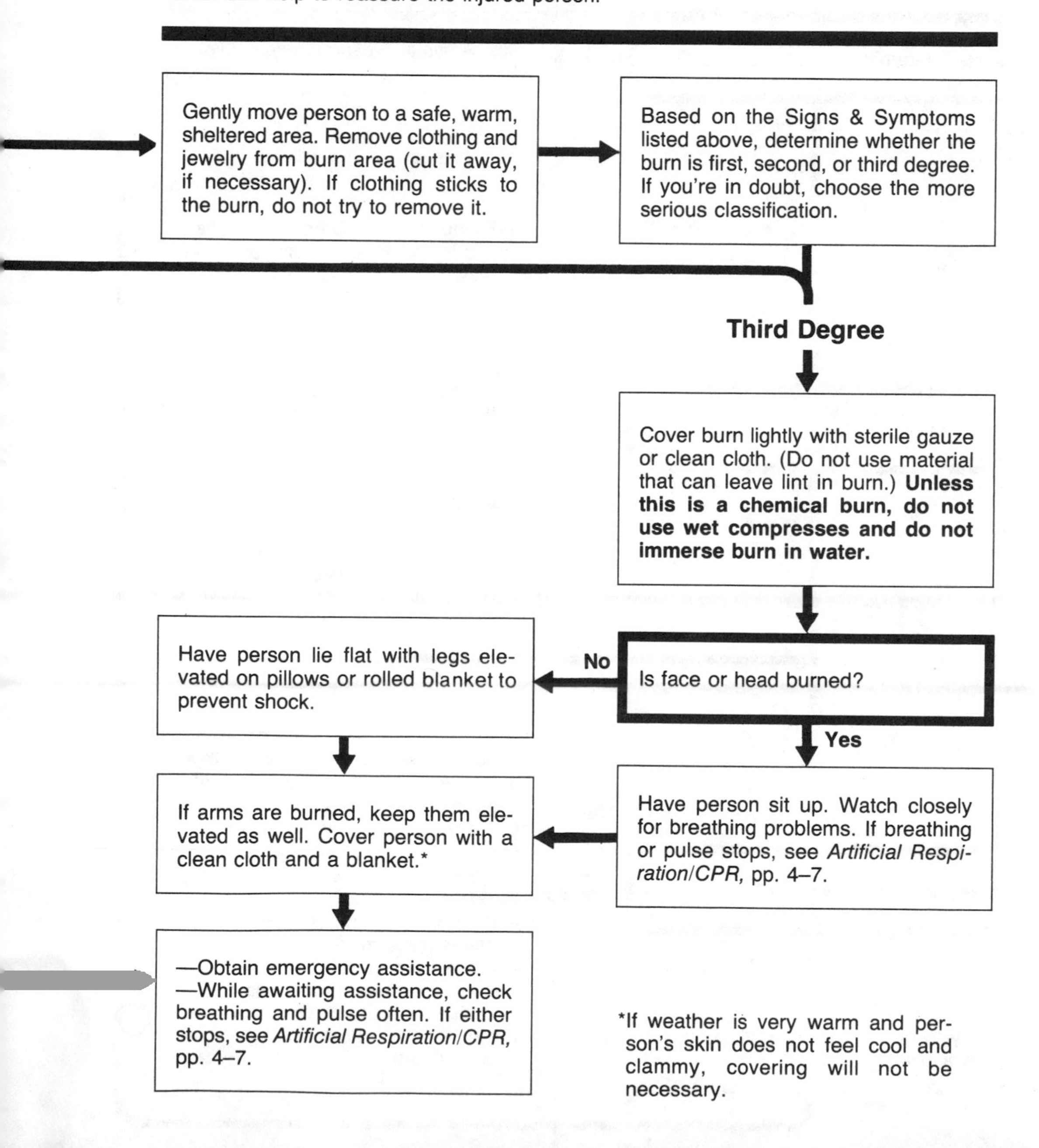
Gently move person to a safe, warm, sheltered area. Remove clothing and jewelry from burn area (cut it away, if necessary). If clothing sticks to the burn, do not try to remove it.
Based on the Signs & Symptoms listed above, determine whether the burn is first, second, or third degree. If you're in doubt, choose the more serious classification.
Third Degree
Cover burn lightly with sterile gauze or clean cloth. (Do not use material that can leave lint in burn.) Unless this is a chemical burn, do not use wet compresses and do not immerse burn in water.
Is face or head burned?
No
Yes
Have person lie flat with legs elevated on pillows or rolled blanket to prevent shock.
Have person sit up. Watch closely for breathing problems. If breathing or pulse stops, see Artificial Respiration/CPR, pp. 4–7.
If arms are burned, keep them elevated as well. Cover person with a clean cloth and a blanket.*
—Obtain emergency assistance.
—While awaiting assistance, check breathing and pulse often. If either stops, see Artificial Respiration/CPR, pp. 4–7.

*If weather is very warm and person's skin does not feel cool and clammy, covering will not be necessary.

Chemical Poisoning

Signs & Symptoms: *an empty container of known poison/sudden onset of abdominal or generalized pain/nausea and vomiting may or may not be present/burns on lips and mouth/distinctive breath odor/stupor or unconsciousness. Symptoms will vary depending on type of poison.*

Contact poison control immediately even if you only suspect poisoning.

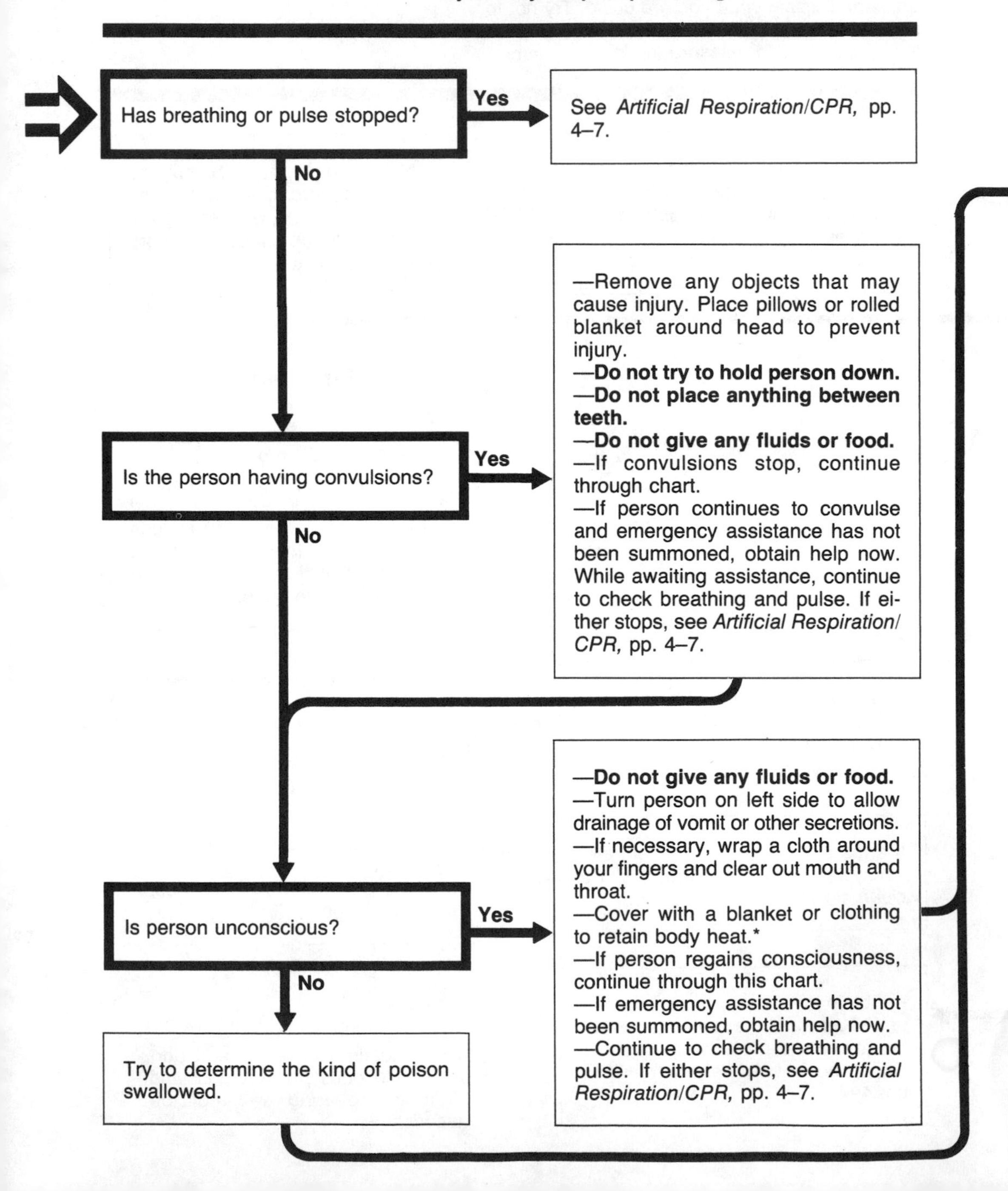

Has breathing or pulse stopped?
Yes
See *Artificial Respiration/CPR,* pp. 4–7.
No
Is the person having convulsions?
Yes
—Remove any objects that may cause injury. Place pillows or rolled blanket around head to prevent injury.
—Do not try to hold person down.
—Do not place anything between teeth.
—Do not give any fluids or food.
—If convulsions stop, continue through chart.
—If person continues to convulse and emergency assistance has not been summoned, obtain help now. While awaiting assistance, continue to check breathing and pulse. If either stops, see *Artificial Respiration/CPR,* pp. 4–7.
No
Is person unconscious?
Yes
—Do not give any fluids or food.
—Turn person on left side to allow drainage of vomit or other secretions.
—If necessary, wrap a cloth around your fingers and clear out mouth and throat.
—Cover with a blanket or clothing to retain body heat.*
—If person regains consciousness, continue through this chart.
—If emergency assistance has not been summoned, obtain help now.
—Continue to check breathing and pulse. If either stops, see *Artificial Respiration/CPR,* pp. 4–7.
No
Try to determine the kind of poison swallowed.

Calm the person by talking while attending to the problem. Explain what you are doing. Try not to show anxiety; act with confidence. Your calm behavior can help reassure the sick person.

If there are two or more rescuers, one should obtain emergency assistance while the other is following the procedures outlined below.

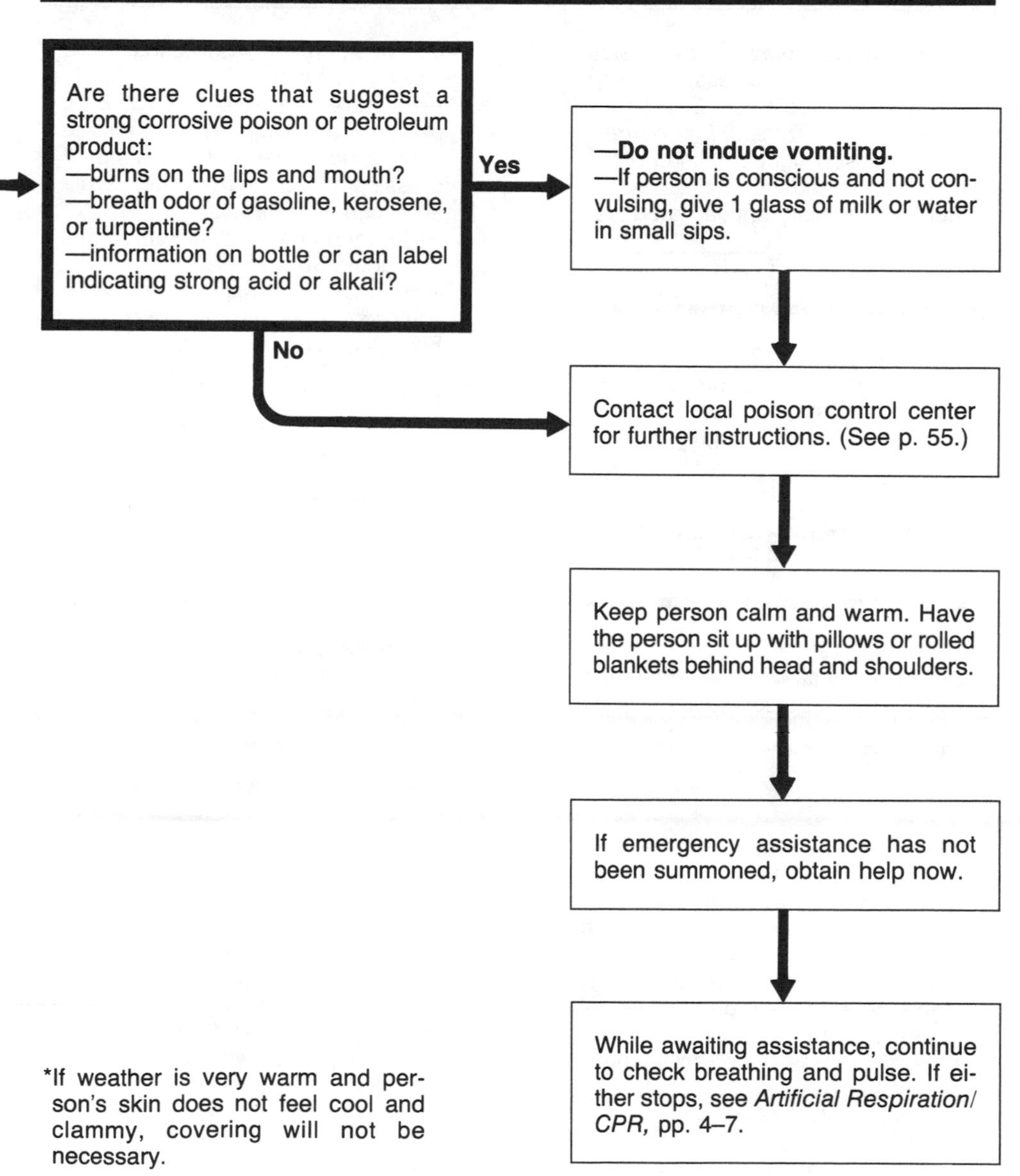
Are there clues that suggest a strong corrosive poison or petroleum product:
—burns on the lips and mouth?
—breath odor of gasoline, kerosene, or turpentine?
—information on bottle or can label indicating strong acid or alkali?
Yes
No
—Do not induce vomiting.
—If person is conscious and not convulsing, give 1 glass of milk or water in small sips.
Contact local poison control center for further instructions. (See p. 55.)
Keep person calm and warm. Have the person sit up with pillows or rolled blankets behind head and shoulders.
If emergency assistance has not been summoned, obtain help now.
While awaiting assistance, continue to check breathing and pulse. If either stops, see Artificial Respiration/CPR, pp. 4–7.

*If weather is very warm and person's skin does not feel cool and clammy, covering will not be necessary.

Chest Injury

For *Chest Pain* without injury, see p. 13.

If there was a severe blow to the head or a fall, or if person is unconscious, assume neck injury and do not move.

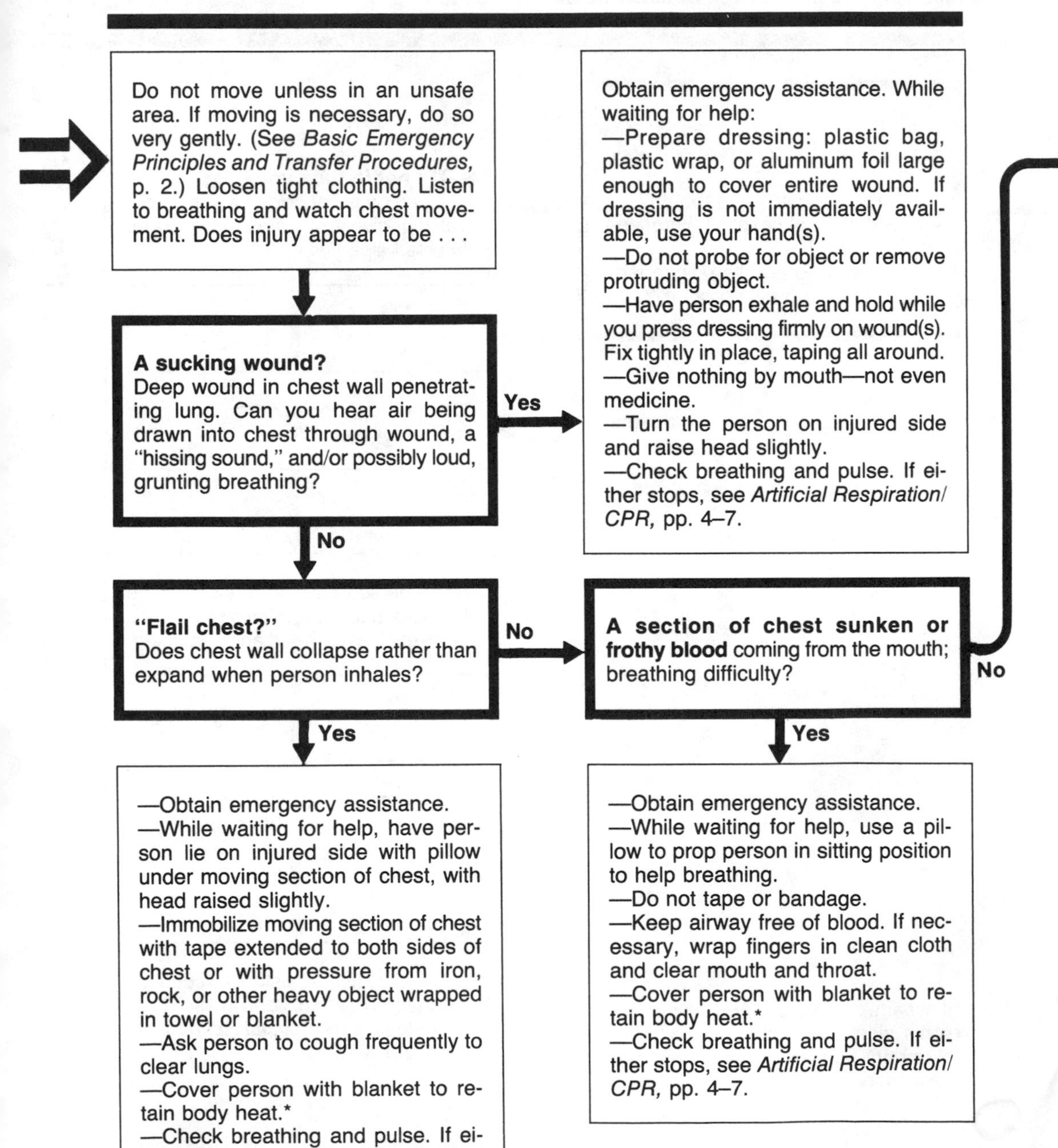

Do not move unless in an unsafe area. If moving is necessary, do so very gently. (See *Basic Emergency Principles and Transfer Procedures,* p. 2.) Loosen tight clothing. Listen to breathing and watch chest movement. Does injury appear to be . . .

A sucking wound?
Deep wound in chest wall penetrating lung. Can you hear air being drawn into chest through wound, a "hissing sound," and/or possibly loud, grunting breathing?

Yes

Obtain emergency assistance. While waiting for help:
—Prepare dressing: plastic bag, plastic wrap, or aluminum foil large enough to cover entire wound. If dressing is not immediately available, use your hand(s).
—Do not probe for object or remove protruding object.
—Have person exhale and hold while you press dressing firmly on wound(s). Fix tightly in place, taping all around.
—Give nothing by mouth—not even medicine.
—Turn the person on injured side and raise head slightly.
—Check breathing and pulse. If either stops, see *Artificial Respiration/CPR,* pp. 4–7.

No

"Flail chest?"
Does chest wall collapse rather than expand when person inhales?

Yes

—Obtain emergency assistance.
—While waiting for help, have person lie on injured side with pillow under moving section of chest, with head raised slightly.
—Immobilize moving section of chest with tape extended to both sides of chest or with pressure from iron, rock, or other heavy object wrapped in towel or blanket.
—Ask person to cough frequently to clear lungs.
—Cover person with blanket to retain body heat.*
—Check breathing and pulse. If either stops, see *Artificial Respiration/CPR,* pp. 4–7.

No

A section of chest sunken or frothy blood coming from the mouth; breathing difficulty?

Yes

—Obtain emergency assistance.
—While waiting for help, use a pillow to prop person in sitting position to help breathing.
—Do not tape or bandage.
—Keep airway free of blood. If necessary, wrap fingers in clean cloth and clear mouth and throat.
—Cover person with blanket to retain body heat.*
—Check breathing and pulse. If either stops, see *Artificial Respiration/CPR,* pp. 4–7.

No

Calm the person by talking while attending to the problem. Explain what you are doing. Try not to show anxiety; act with confidence. Your calm behavior can help to reassure the injured person.

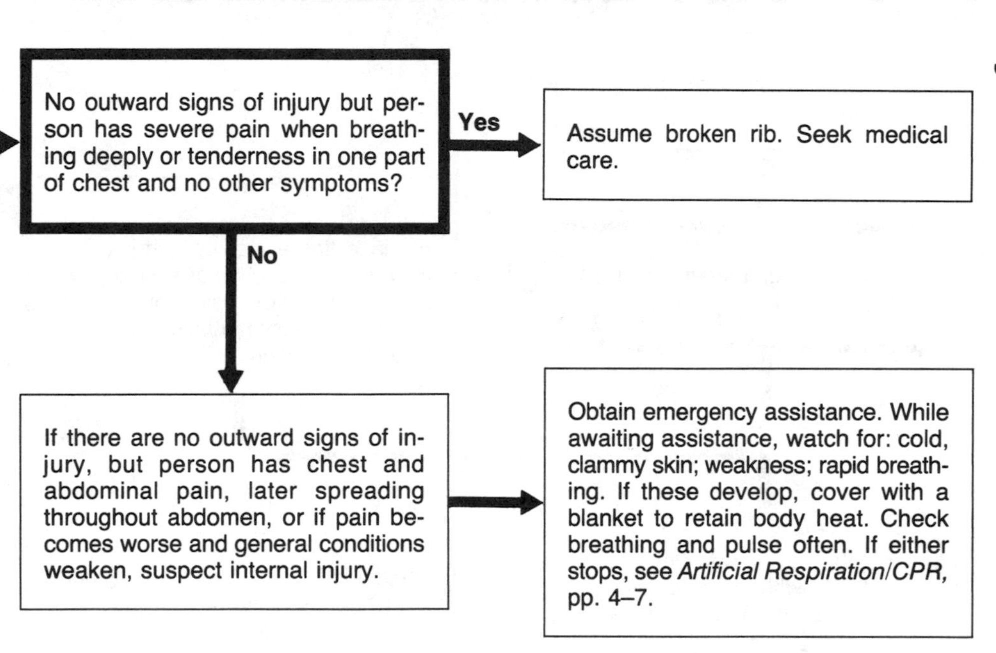
No outward signs of injury but person has severe pain when breathing deeply or tenderness in one part of chest and no other symptoms?
Yes
Assume broken rib. Seek medical care.
No
If there are no outward signs of injury, but person has chest and abdominal pain, later spreading throughout abdomen, or if pain becomes worse and general conditions weaken, suspect internal injury.
Obtain emergency assistance. While awaiting assistance, watch for: cold, clammy skin; weakness; rapid breathing. If these develop, cover with a blanket to retain body heat. Check breathing and pulse often. If either stops, see *Artificial Respiration/CPR,* pp. 4–7.

*If weather is very warm and person's skin does not feel cool and clammy, covering will not be necessary.

34 Minor Cuts
(Including Rope Burns)

Definition: *minor bleeding/no involvement of underlying tissue (nerve, muscle, tendon, artery, vein)*

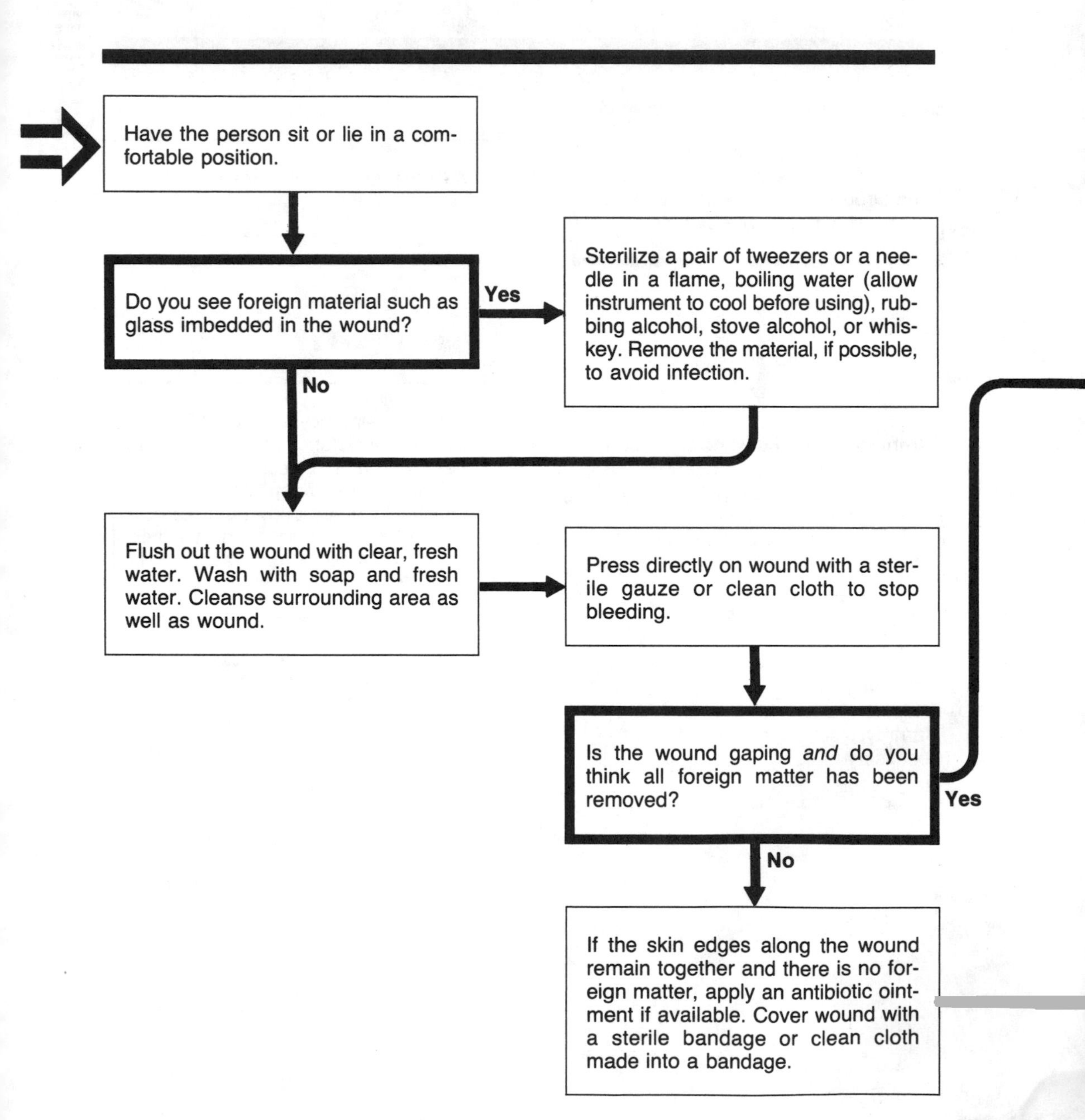

Have the person sit or lie in a comfortable position.
Do you see foreign material such as glass imbedded in the wound?
Yes
Sterilize a pair of tweezers or a needle in a flame, boiling water (allow instrument to cool before using), rubbing alcohol, stove alcohol, or whiskey. Remove the material, if possible, to avoid infection.
No
Flush out the wound with clear, fresh water. Wash with soap and fresh water. Cleanse surrounding area as well as wound.
Press directly on wound with a sterile gauze or clean cloth to stop bleeding.
Is the wound gaping *and* do you think all foreign matter has been removed?
Yes
No
If the skin edges along the wound remain together and there is no foreign matter, apply an antibiotic ointment if available. Cover wound with a sterile bandage or clean cloth made into a bandage.

Calm the person by talking while attending to the problem. Explain what you are doing. Try not to show anxiety; act with confidence. Your calm behavior can help to reassure the injured person.

If injury was the result of a vehicular or job-related accident, the person should be examined by a physician for possible additional injuries or complications.

Form a butterfly strip from adhesive tape. Draw the skin edges together and use the strips to close the wound. No other dressing should be necessary unless wound is on foot, then pad with gauze and tape in place.

Seek medical care as soon as possible. Person may require sutures and/or tetanus immunization.

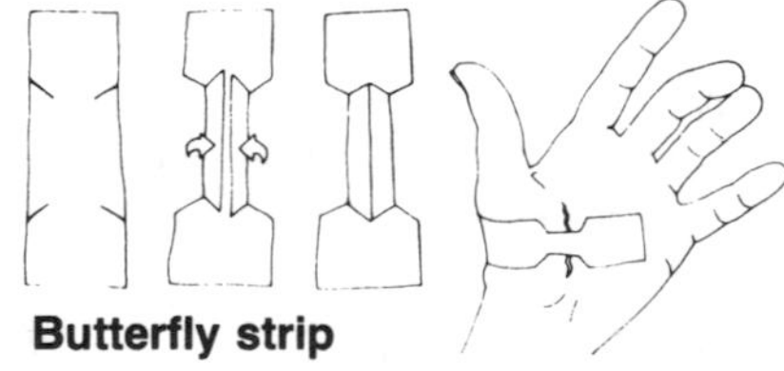

Butterfly strip

Take a strip of adhesive tape about 3½ inches long . . . Make four cuts (slightly inward) and fold in, sticky side to sticky side.

If person has not received tetanus shot within 5 years, if wound is very dirty or has foreign matter, or if any signs of infection develop (redness, swelling, etc.), seek medical care.

35 Dislocations

Signs & Symptoms: *distortion in a shape of joint/ swelling and discoloration/pain with movement/ affected limb looks longer or shorter/loss of movement in joint.*

If you suspect *Back or Neck Injury*, see p. 29.
If you suspect a *Fracture*, see p. 41.

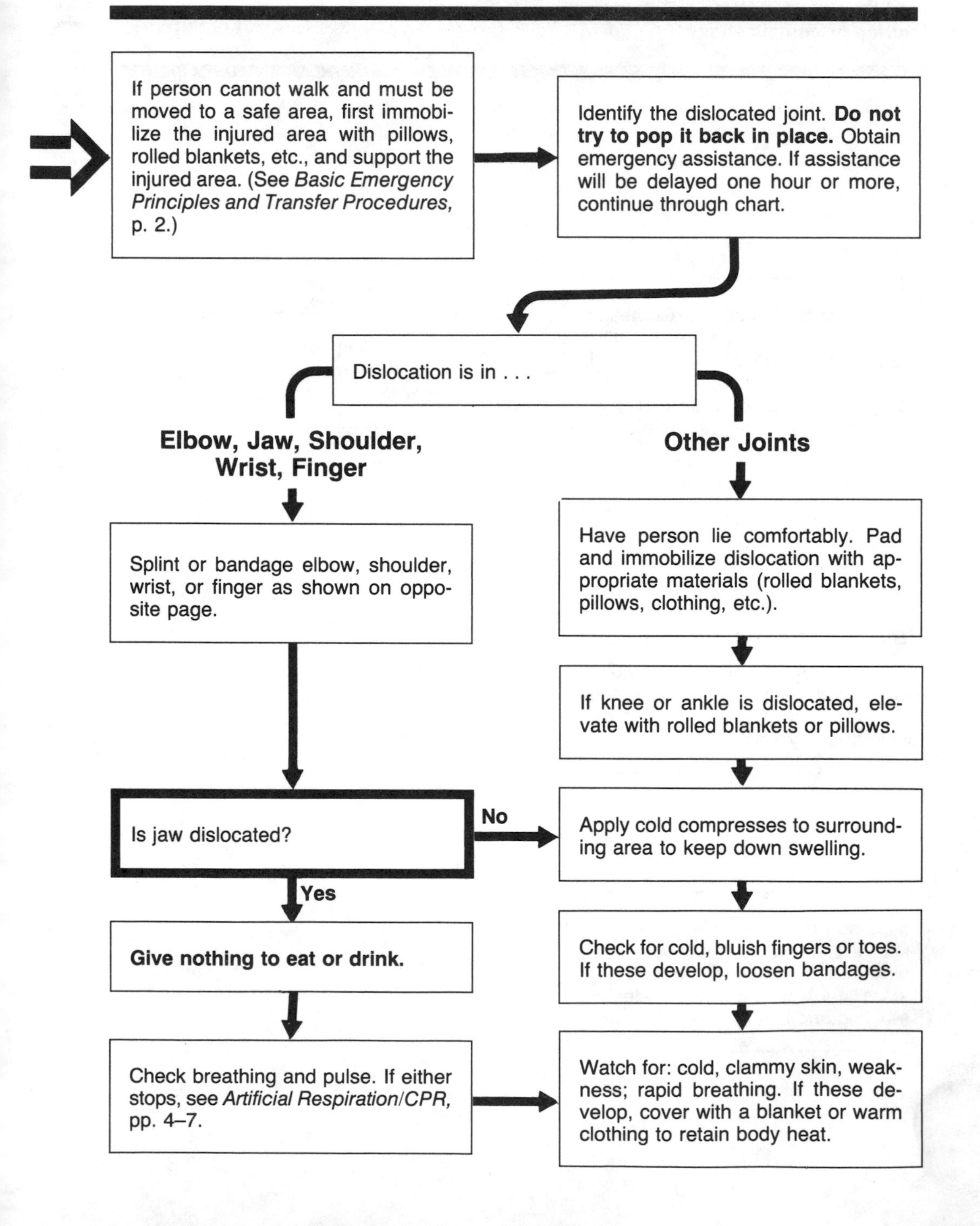
If person cannot walk and must be moved to a safe area, first immobilize the injured area with pillows, rolled blankets, etc., and support the injured area. (See *Basic Emergency Principles and Transfer Procedures,* p. 2.)
Identify the dislocated joint. **Do not try to pop it back in place.** Obtain emergency assistance. If assistance will be delayed one hour or more, continue through chart.
Dislocation is in . . .
Elbow, Jaw, Shoulder, Wrist, Finger
Other Joints
Splint or bandage elbow, shoulder, wrist, or finger as shown on opposite page.
Have person lie comfortably. Pad and immobilize dislocation with appropriate materials (rolled blankets, pillows, clothing, etc.).
If knee or ankle is dislocated, elevate with rolled blankets or pillows.
Is jaw dislocated?
No
Apply cold compresses to surrounding area to keep down swelling.
Yes
Give nothing to eat or drink.
Check for cold, bluish fingers or toes. If these develop, loosen bandages.
Check breathing and pulse. If either stops, see *Artificial Respiration/CPR,* pp. 4–7.
Watch for: cold, clammy skin, weakness; rapid breathing. If these develop, cover with a blanket or warm clothing to retain body heat.

Calm the person by talking while attending to the problem. Explain what you are doing. Try not to show anxiety; act with confidence. Your calm behavior can help to reassure the injured person.

Finger

splints: eating spoons, padded stick, other finger.

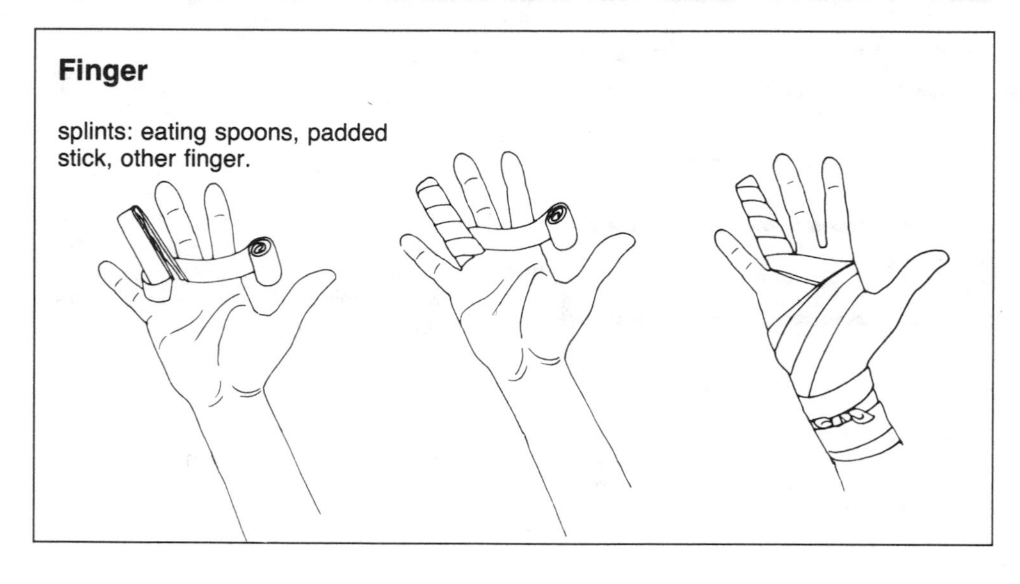

Elbow, Shoulder, or Wrist Sling

suggested materials:
shirt or jacket,
large handkerchief, towel, bandanna,
or piece of sheet folded diagonally.

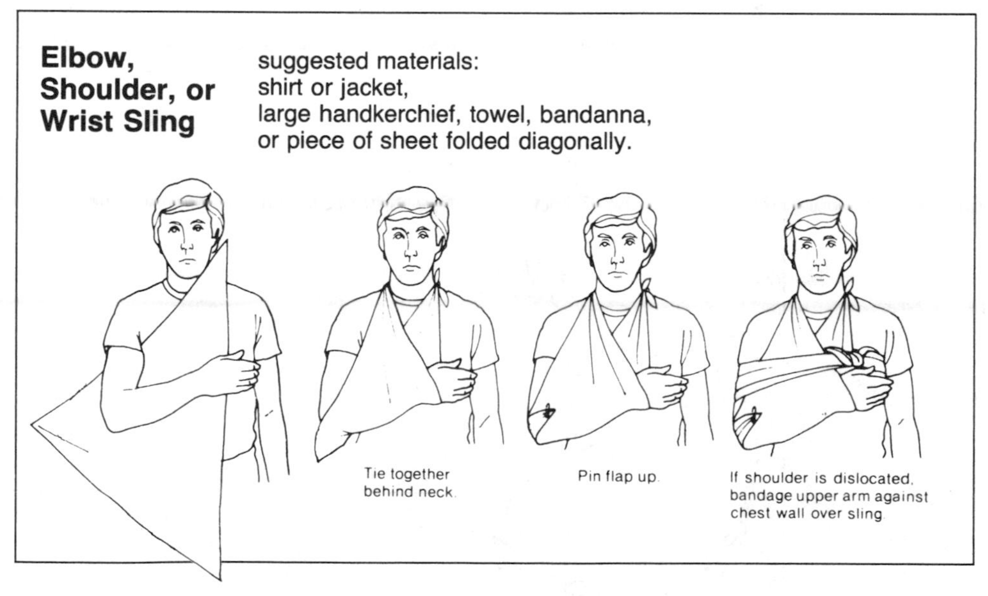

Tie together behind neck.

Pin flap up.

If shoulder is dislocated, bandage upper arm against chest wall over sling.

36 Chemical Burns of the Eyes

If there are two or more rescuers, one should obtain emergency assistance while the other is following the procedures outlined below.

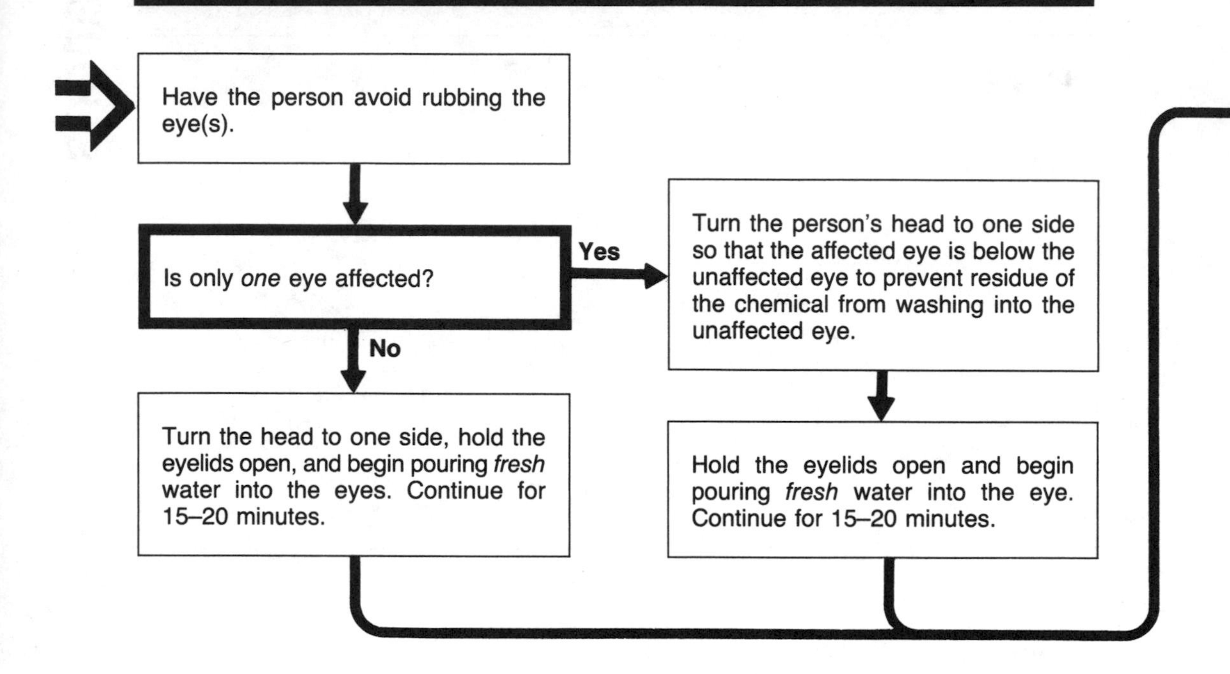

Have the person avoid rubbing the eye(s).
Is only *one* eye affected?
Yes
Turn the person's head to one side so that the affected eye is below the unaffected eye to prevent residue of the chemical from washing into the unaffected eye.
Hold the eyelids open and begin pouring *fresh* water into the eye. Continue for 15–20 minutes.
No
Turn the head to one side, hold the eyelids open, and begin pouring *fresh* water into the eyes. Continue for 15–20 minutes.

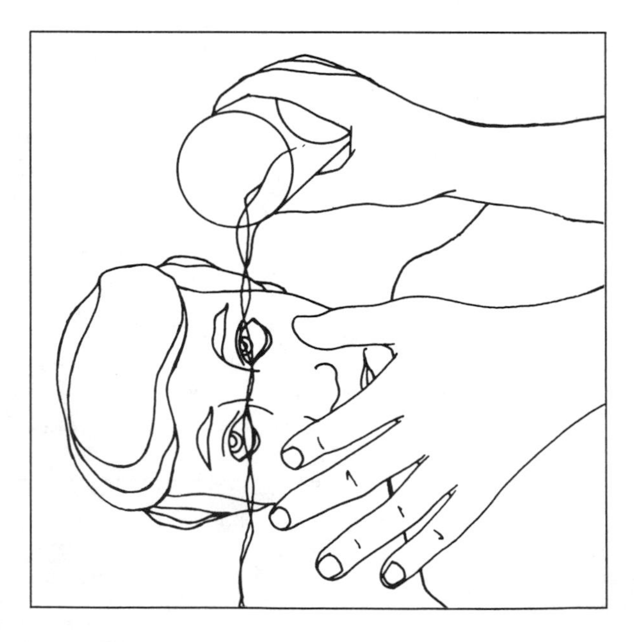

Calm the person by talking while attending to the problem. Explain what you are doing. Try not to show anxiety; act with confidence. Your calm behavior can help to reassure the injured person.

Remove the coagulated chemical from the eye with moistened sterile gauze.

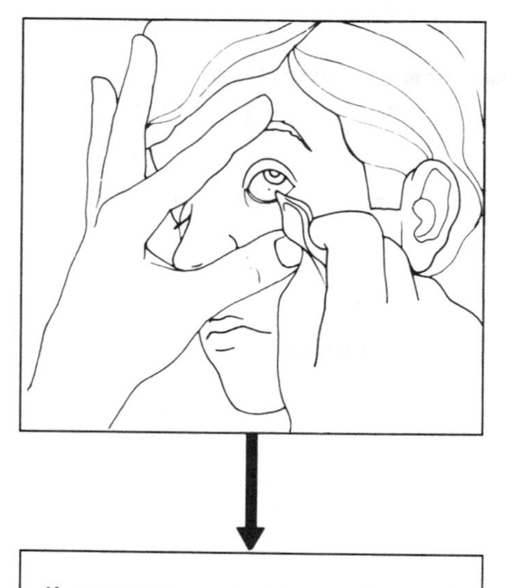

If emergency assistance has not been summoned, obtain help now.

While awaiting assistance, continue to rinse out the eye(s) until help arrives.

37 Foreign Object in Eye

(With no injury or bleeding)

For chemicals in eye, see *Chemical Burns of the Eyes,* p. 36.

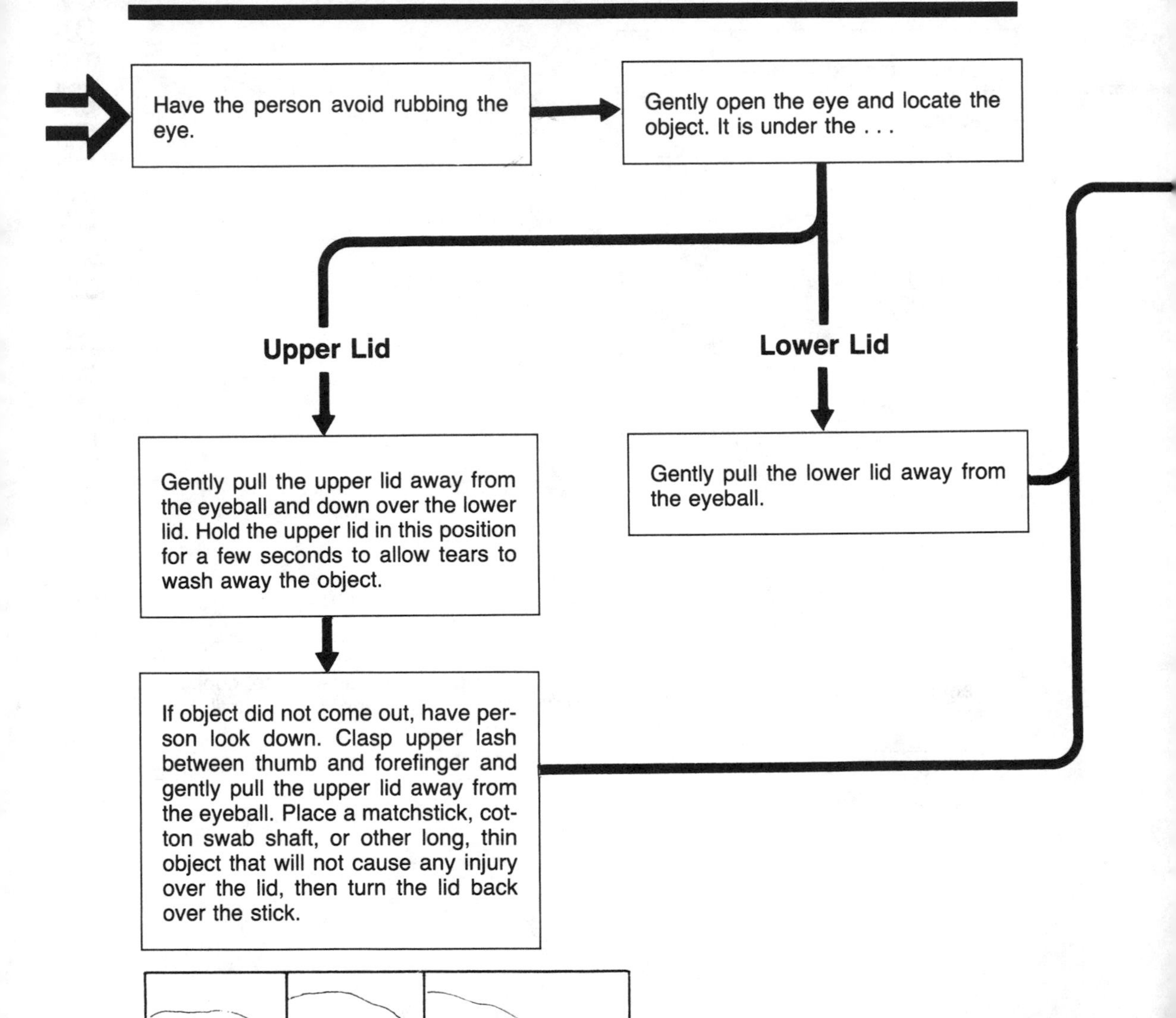

Have the person avoid rubbing the eye.

Gently open the eye and locate the object. It is under the . . .

Upper Lid

Gently pull the upper lid away from the eyeball and down over the lower lid. Hold the upper lid in this position for a few seconds to allow tears to wash away the object.

If object did not come out, have person look down. Clasp upper lash between thumb and forefinger and gently pull the upper lid away from the eyeball. Place a matchstick, cotton swab shaft, or other long, thin object that will not cause any injury over the lid, then turn the lid back over the stick.

Lower Lid

Gently pull the lower lid away from the eyeball.

Calm the person by talking while attending to the problem. Explain what you are doing. Try not to show anxiety; act with confidence. Your calm behavior can help to reassure the injured person.

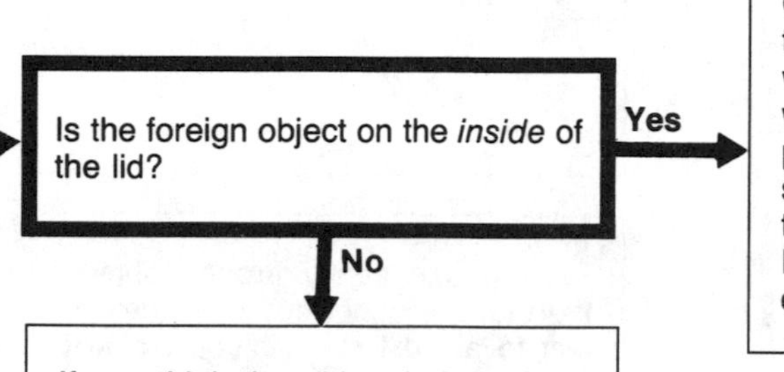
Is the foreign object on the *inside* of the lid?
Yes
No

Gently remove it with a moistened tissue or cloth or by pouring fresh water in eye. No further treatment will be necessary unless swelling, pain, discoloration, or change in vision develop or if there is a sensation that something is still in the eye. If any of these occur, seek medical care.

If you think the object is imbedded in the cornea, do not attempt to remove it. Cover both eyes with a dry bandage. **Do not apply any pressure.** Seek medical care.

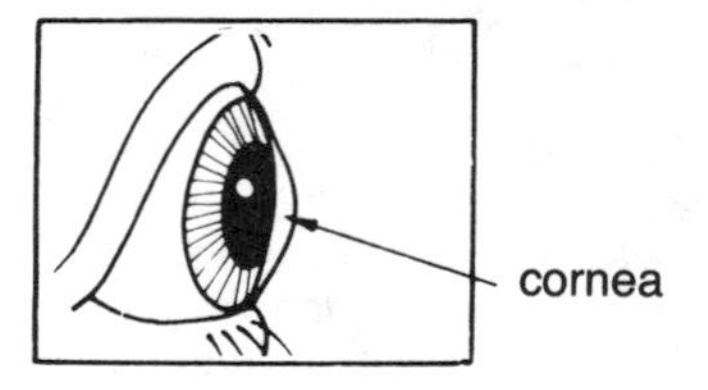
cornea

Eye Injury

For chemicals in the eye, see p. 36. For small foreign object in eye, but not penetrating eye, see p. 37.

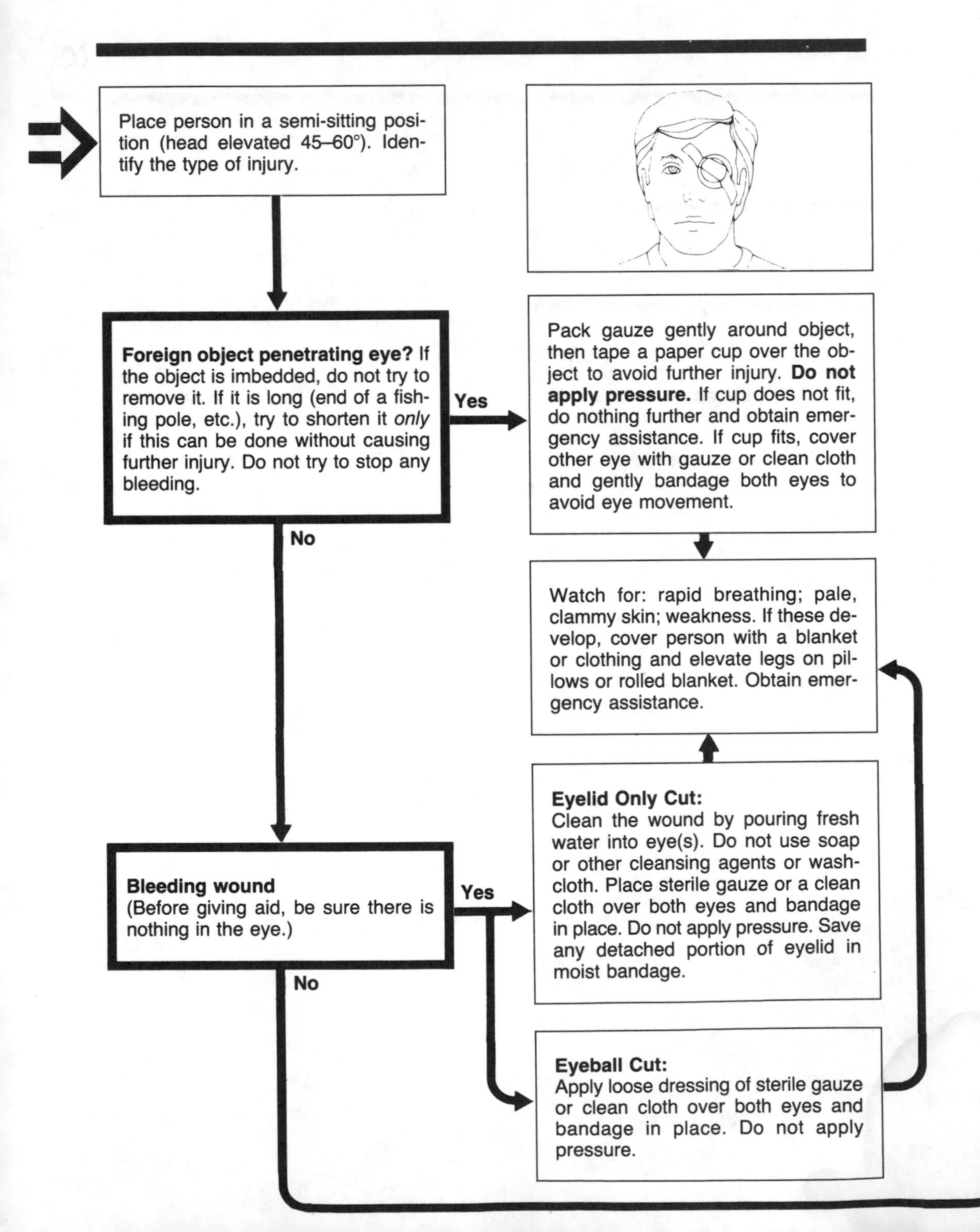

Place person in a semi-sitting position (head elevated 45–60°). Identify the type of injury.
Foreign object penetrating eye? If the object is imbedded, do not try to remove it. If it is long (end of a fishing pole, etc.), try to shorten it only if this can be done without causing further injury. Do not try to stop any bleeding.
Yes
Pack gauze gently around object, then tape a paper cup over the object to avoid further injury. Do not apply pressure. If cup does not fit, do nothing further and obtain emergency assistance. If cup fits, cover other eye with gauze or clean cloth and gently bandage both eyes to avoid eye movement.
Watch for: rapid breathing; pale, clammy skin; weakness. If these develop, cover person with a blanket or clothing and elevate legs on pillows or rolled blanket. Obtain emergency assistance.
No
Bleeding wound
(Before giving aid, be sure there is nothing in the eye.)
Yes
Eyelid Only Cut:
Clean the wound by pouring fresh water into eye(s). Do not use soap or other cleansing agents or washcloth. Place sterile gauze or a clean cloth over both eyes and bandage in place. Do not apply pressure. Save any detached portion of eyelid in moist bandage.
Eyeball Cut:
Apply loose dressing of sterile gauze or clean cloth over both eyes and bandage in place. Do not apply pressure.
No

Calm the person by talking while attending to the problem. Explain what you are doing. Try not to show anxiety; act with confidence. Your calm behavior can help to reassure the injured person.

If injury was the result of a vehicular or job-related accident, the person should be examined by a physician for possible additional injuries or complications.

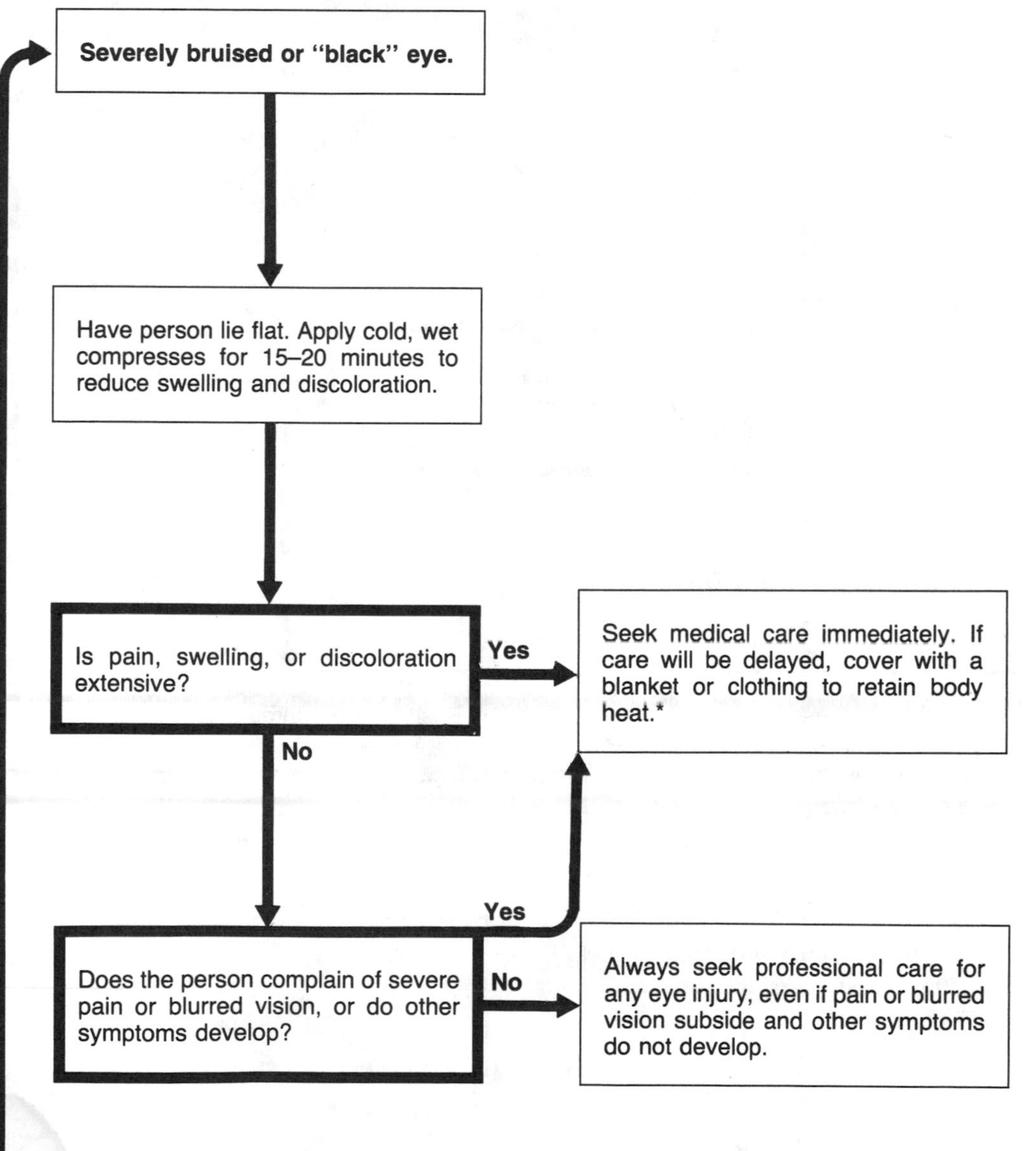
Severely bruised or "black" eye.
Have person lie flat. Apply cold, wet compresses for 15–20 minutes to reduce swelling and discoloration.
Is pain, swelling, or discoloration extensive?
Yes
No
Seek medical care immediately. If care will be delayed, cover with a blanket or clothing to retain body heat.*
Does the person complain of severe pain or blurred vision, or do other symptoms develop?
Yes
No
Always seek professional care for any eye injury, even if pain or blurred vision subside and other symptoms do not develop.

*If weather is very warm and person's skin does not feel cool and clammy, covering will not be necessary.

39 Fishhook Removal

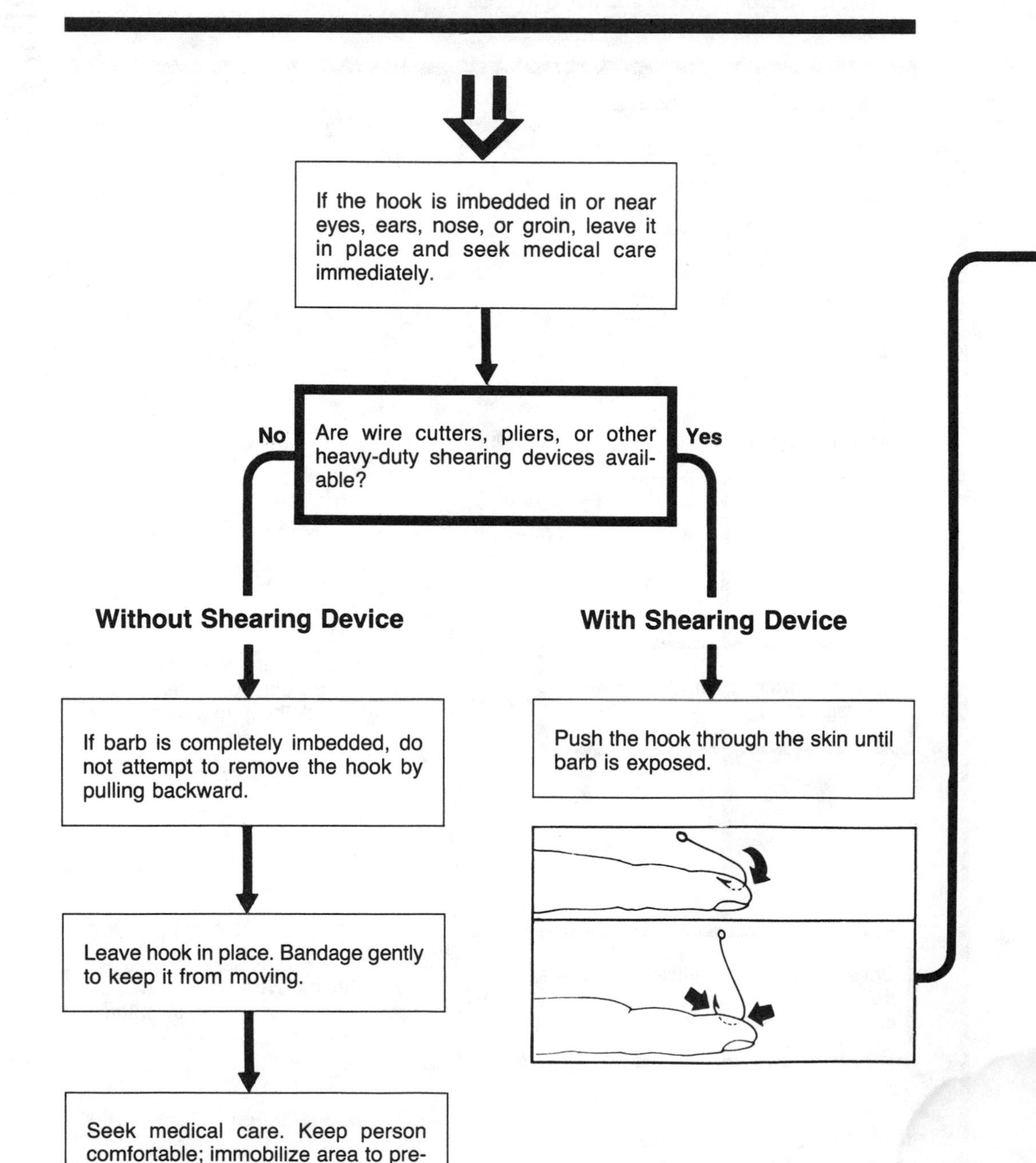
If the hook is imbedded in or near eyes, ears, nose, or groin, leave it in place and seek medical care immediately.
Are wire cutters, pliers, or other heavy-duty shearing devices available?
No
Yes
Without Shearing Device
With Shearing Device
If barb is completely imbedded, do not attempt to remove the hook by pulling backward.
Leave hook in place. Bandage gently to keep it from moving.
Seek medical care. Keep person comfortable; immobilize area to prevent further injury.
Push the hook through the skin until barb is exposed.

Calm the person by talking while attending to the problem. Explain what you are doing. Try not to show anxiety; act with confidence. Your calm behavior can help to reassure the injured person.

Carefully cover the area with a cloth or towel to avoid being hit by a piece of the hook when it is cut. Cut the shank of the hook at the base of the barb and remove the pieces.

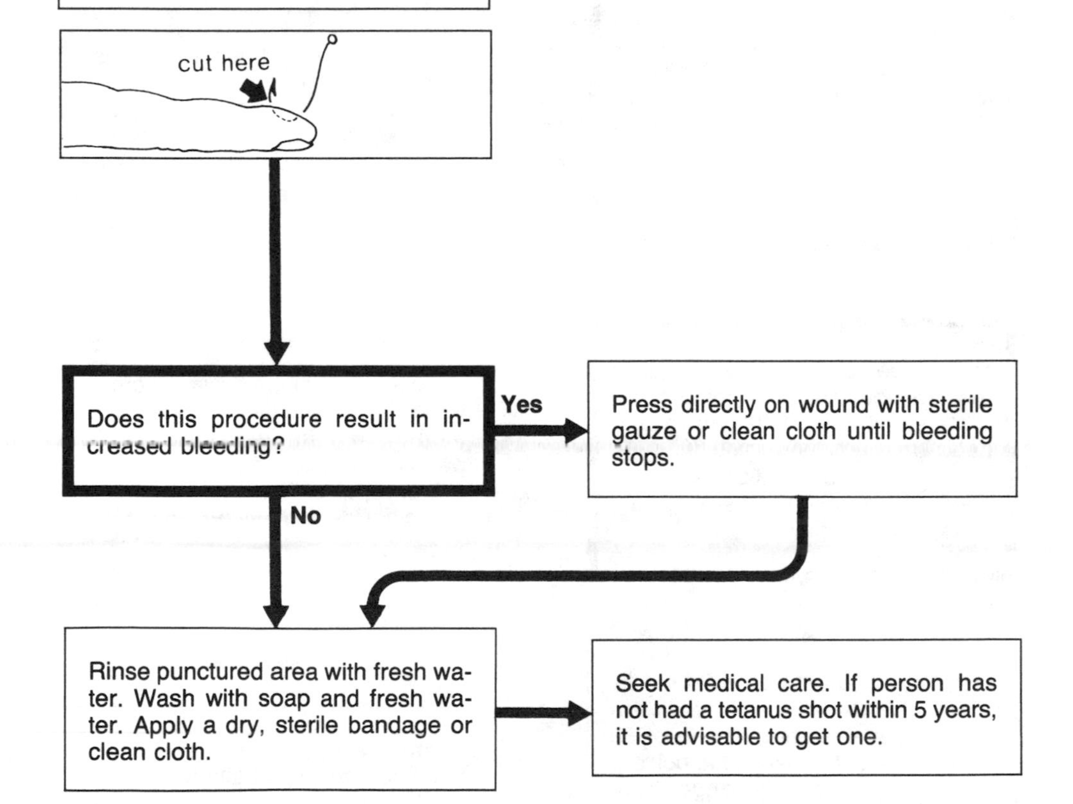
cut here

Does this procedure result in increased bleeding?

Yes → Press directly on wound with sterile gauze or clean cloth until bleeding stops.

No → Rinse punctured area with fresh water. Wash with soap and fresh water. Apply a dry, sterile bandage or clean cloth.

Seek medical care. If person has not had a tetanus shot within 5 years, it is advisable to get one.

Food Poisoning

If there are two or more rescuers, one should obtain emergency assistance while the other is following the procedures outlined below.

Signs & Symptoms: *nausea/possible vomiting/chills/diarrhea/cramps/recent ingestion of food that "didn't taste right" or was old or otherwise suspect/others with same symptoms. See other symptoms in chart.*

For food allergy, see *Allergic Reaction*, p. 27.

If the person is conscious, has not vomited, and there is no convulsion or difficulty swallowing or breathing, give milk or water. If person is vomiting, save the vomitus for evaluation.

Has the person eaten home-canned vegetables or smoked meats within last 12–36 hours and are the symptoms muscle weakness, headache, dizziness, slurred speech, disturbed vision, breathing or swallowing difficulty, or coma?

Yes → Suspect botulism. If emergency assistance has not been summoned, obtain help now. While awaiting assistance, check breathing and pulse. If either stops, see *Artificial Respiration/CPR,* pp. 4–7.

No ↓

Has the person eaten shellfish within the last hour and do symptoms include numbness around face and head gradually spreading throughout entire body, dizziness, increased salivation, muscle weakness, or paralysis?

Yes → Suspect shellfish poisoning. If emergency assistance has not been summoned, obtain help now. While awaiting assistance, check breathing and pulse. If either stops, see *Artificial Respiration/CPR,* pp. 4–7.

No ↓

If the person has eaten wild mushrooms, berries, plants, other suspicious foods or water within past 12 hours, suspect general food poisoning. Symptoms can range from nausea, vomiting, and cramps to hallucinations or slurred speech.

→ If emergency assistance has not been summoned, obtain help now.

Calm the person by talking while attending to the problem. Explain what you are doing. Try not to show anxiety; act with confidence. Your calm behavior can help to reassure the sick person.

Contact local poison control center for further instructions. (See p. 55.)

If unable to reach poison control center, give medicinal activated charcoal powder, 30 grams in 6 ounces of water.

While awaiting assistance, make person comfortable. Have person lie on side and cover with a blanket or clothing to retain body heat.*

Watch for choking and keep airway clear. If necessary, wrap cloth around fingers to clear vomit from throat. Send sample of vomitus and food container for evaluation.

*If weather is very warm and person's skin does not feel cool and clammy, covering will not be necessary.

Fractures

For *Severe Head Injury*, see p. 42.
For *Back and Neck Injuries*, see p. 29.

Signs & Symptoms: *sound of bone snapping/deformity with swelling and discoloration/painful to touch/possible grating sensation of broken bone ends. With any injury, if you're not sure, assume there is a fracture.*

If there are two or more rescuers, one should obtain emergency assistance while the other is following the procedures outlined below.

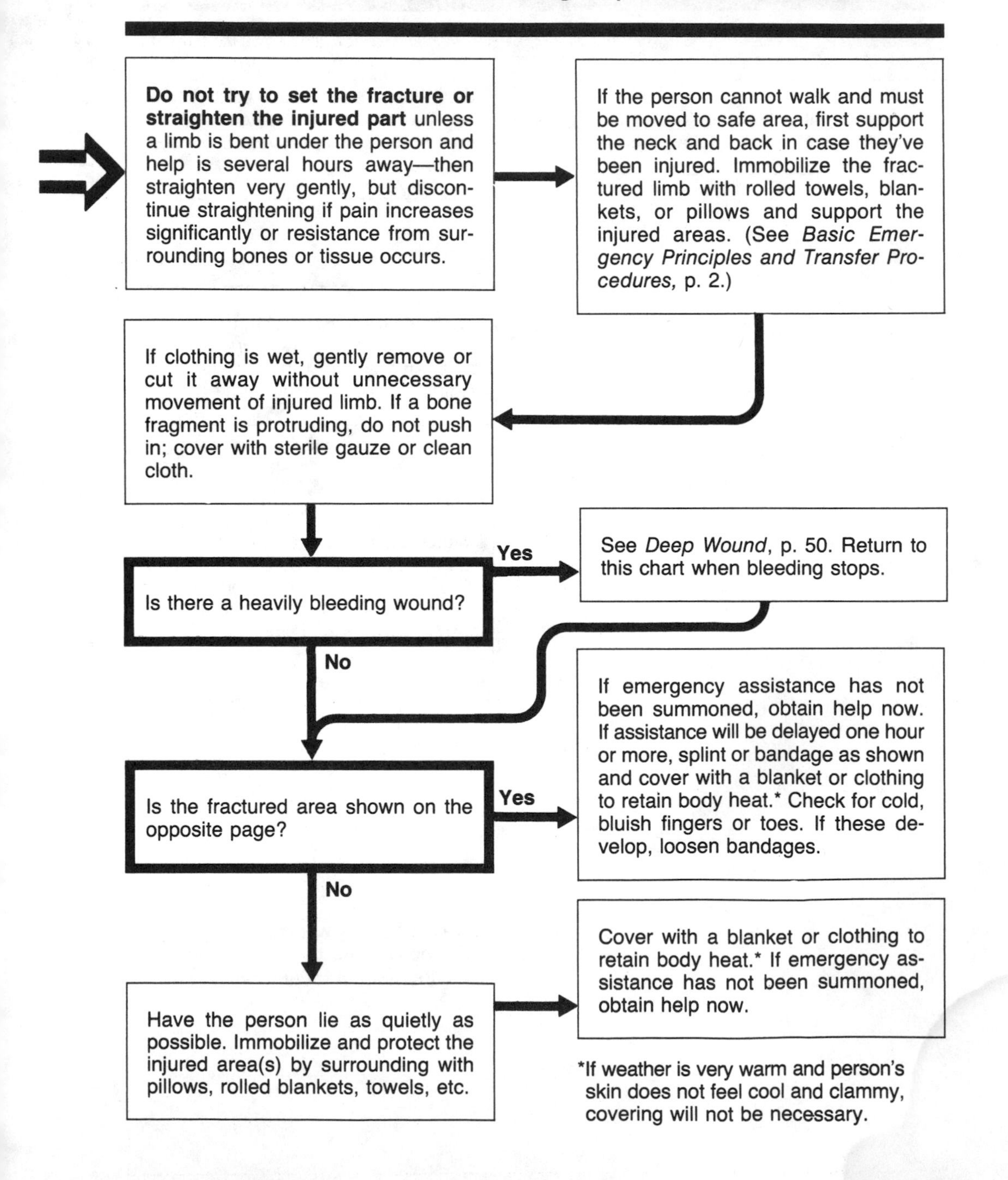
Do not try to set the fracture or straighten the injured part unless a limb is bent under the person and help is several hours away—then straighten very gently, but discontinue straightening if pain increases significantly or resistance from surrounding bones or tissue occurs.
If the person cannot walk and must be moved to safe area, first support the neck and back in case they've been injured. Immobilize the fractured limb with rolled towels, blankets, or pillows and support the injured areas. (See Basic Emergency Principles and Transfer Procedures, p. 2.)
If clothing is wet, gently remove or cut it away without unnecessary movement of injured limb. If a bone fragment is protruding, do not push in; cover with sterile gauze or clean cloth.
Is there a heavily bleeding wound?
Yes
See Deep Wound, p. 50. Return to this chart when bleeding stops.
No
Is the fractured area shown on the opposite page?
Yes
If emergency assistance has not been summoned, obtain help now. If assistance will be delayed one hour or more, splint or bandage as shown and cover with a blanket or clothing to retain body heat.* Check for cold, bluish fingers or toes. If these develop, loosen bandages.
No
Have the person lie as quietly as possible. Immobilize and protect the injured area(s) by surrounding with pillows, rolled blankets, towels, etc.
Cover with a blanket or clothing to retain body heat.* If emergency assistance has not been summoned, obtain help now.
*If weather is very warm and person's skin does not feel cool and clammy, covering will not be necessary.

Calm the person by talking while attending to the problem. Explain what you are doing. Try not to show anxiety; act with confidence. Your calm behavior can help to reassure the injured person.

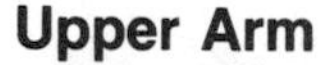

Upper Arm

Splints: rolled magazines, newspapers, or heavy cardboard; cooking spoons, garden stakes, or tool handles wrapped in sheeting, towels, or shirts for padding. Sling: sheeting, large handkerchief, or towel folded diagonally.

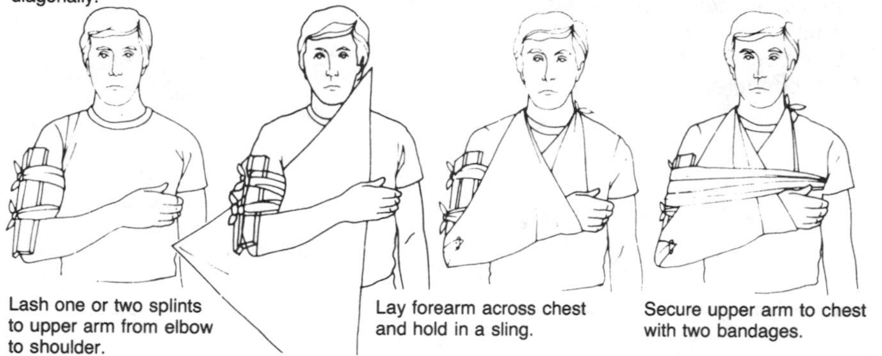

Lash one or two splints to upper arm from elbow to shoulder.

Lay forearm across chest and hold in a sling.

Secure upper arm to chest with two bandages.

Forearm, wrist, or hand

Use rolled handkerchief as pad to be grasped in hand, then splint as for upper arm and put in sling.

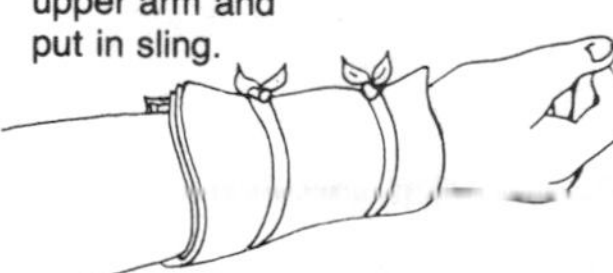

Elbow splint

Suggested materials for splint: Same as for upper arm.

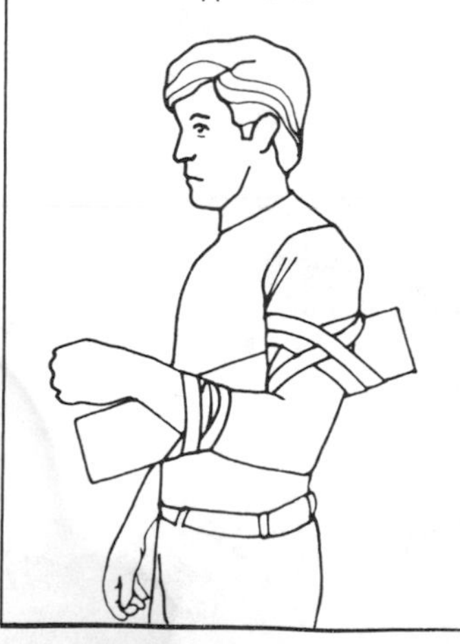

Collarbone

Make sling and secure as shown.

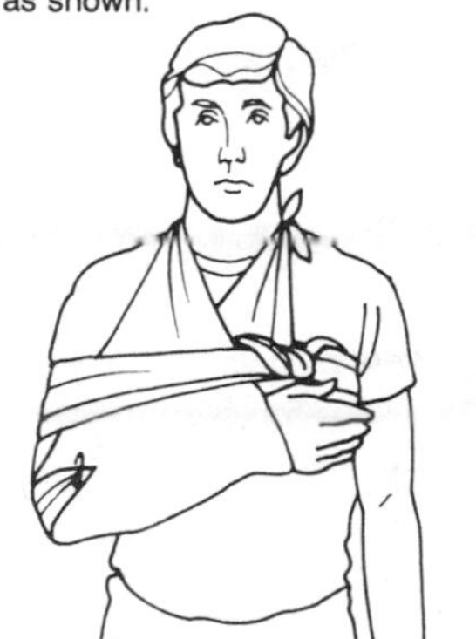

Ankle and Foot

Pad injured part firmly with blanket, towels, or pillow. Secure with tape or strips of cloth. Keep leg elevated.

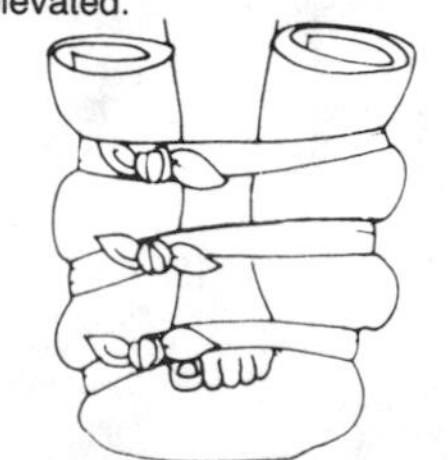

Finger

Splints: eating spoon, padded stick, other finger.

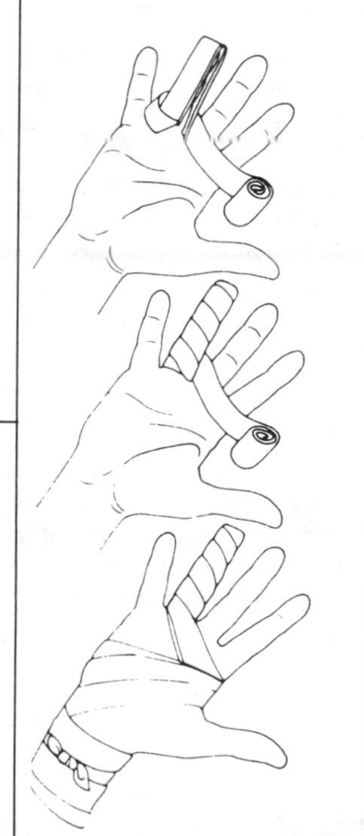

Severe Head Injury

Signs & Symptoms

Skull fracture: *dizziness/double vision/slurred speech/headache/possible bleeding or draining of clear fluid from ears, nose, or mouth/possible nausea and vomiting/possible convulsions/pupils of unequal size/paralysis on the side opposite injury/deformity of skull/unconsciousness. One eye may appear sunken.*

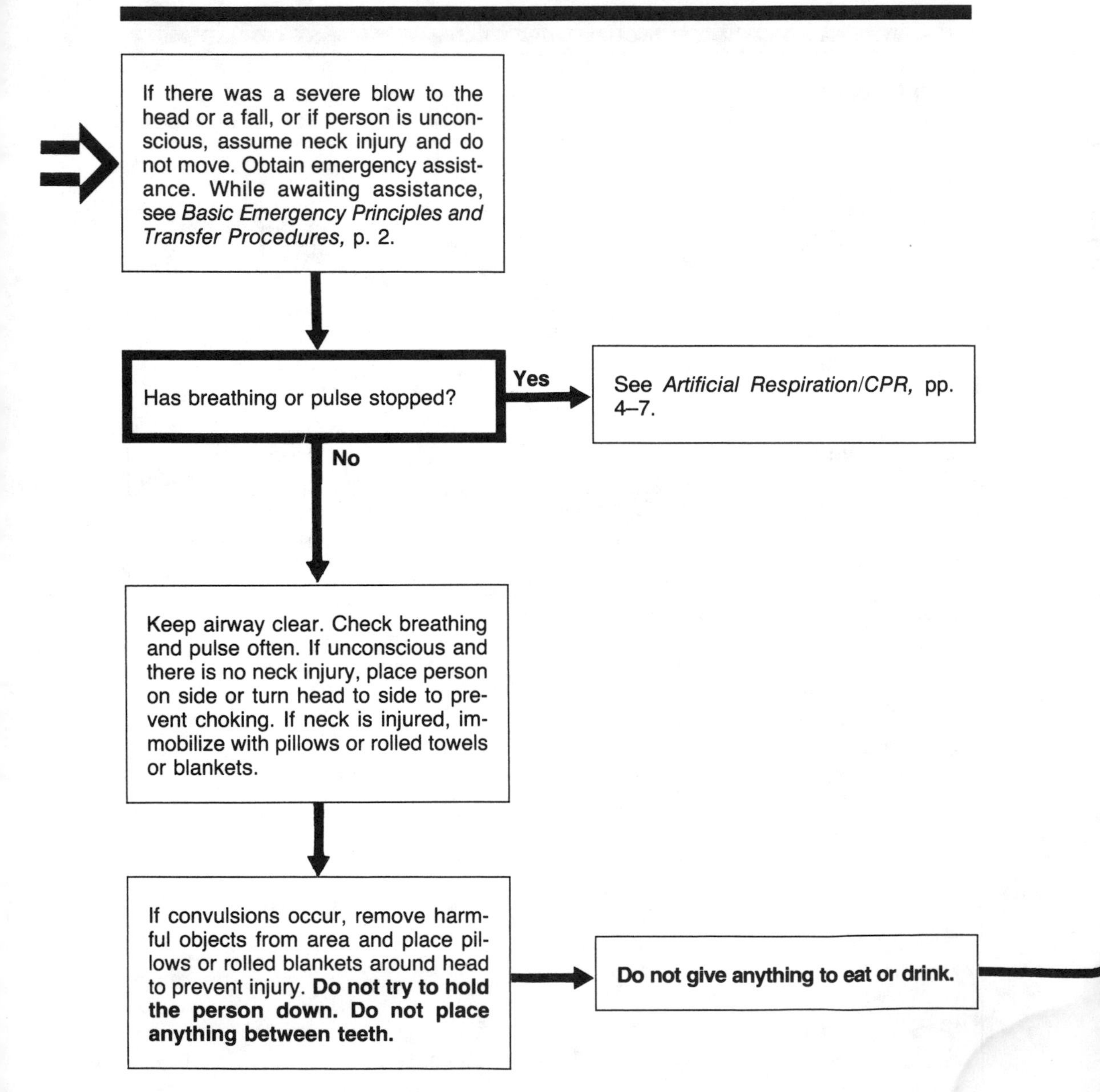

If there was a severe blow to the head or a fall, or if person is unconscious, assume neck injury and do not move. Obtain emergency assistance. While awaiting assistance, see *Basic Emergency Principles and Transfer Procedures,* p. 2.
Has breathing or pulse stopped?
Yes
See *Artificial Respiration/CPR,* pp. 4–7.
No
Keep airway clear. Check breathing and pulse often. If unconscious and there is no neck injury, place person on side or turn head to side to prevent choking. If neck is injured, immobilize with pillows or rolled towels or blankets.
If convulsions occur, remove harmful objects from area and place pillows or rolled blankets around head to prevent injury. **Do not try to hold the person down. Do not place anything between teeth.**
Do not give anything to eat or drink.

Calm the person by talking while attending to the problem. Explain what you are doing. Try not to show anxiety; act with confidence. Your calm behavior can help to reassure the injured person.

If there are two or more rescuers, one should obtain emergency assistance while the other is following the procedures outlined below.

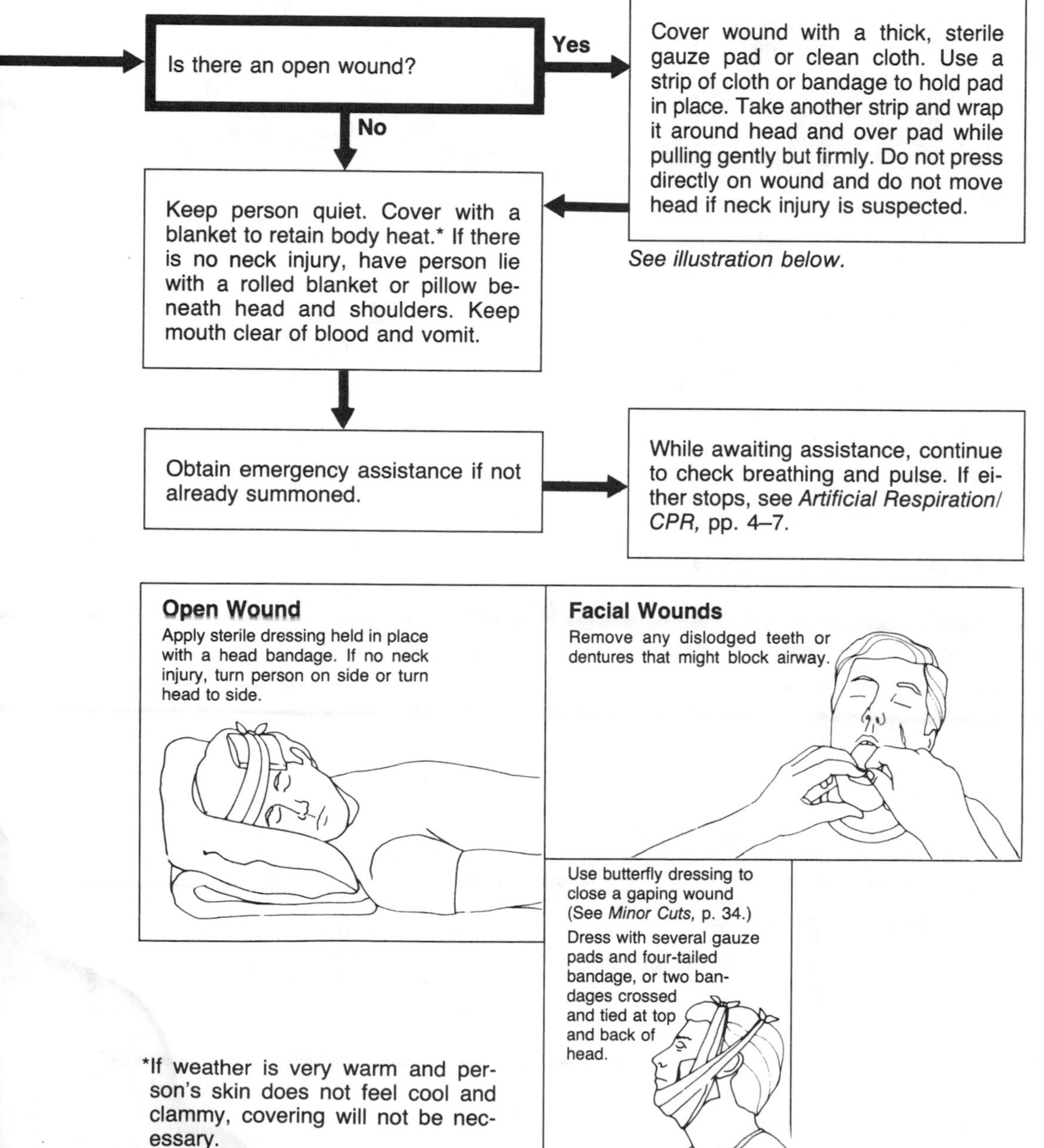
Is there an open wound?
Yes
Cover wound with a thick, sterile gauze pad or clean cloth. Use a strip of cloth or bandage to hold pad in place. Take another strip and wrap it around head and over pad while pulling gently but firmly. Do not press directly on wound and do not move head if neck injury is suspected.
See illustration below.
No
Keep person quiet. Cover with a blanket to retain body heat.* If there is no neck injury, have person lie with a rolled blanket or pillow beneath head and shoulders. Keep mouth clear of blood and vomit.
Obtain emergency assistance if not already summoned.
While awaiting assistance, continue to check breathing and pulse. If either stops, see Artificial Respiration/CPR, pp. 4–7.
Open Wound
Apply sterile dressing held in place with a head bandage. If no neck injury, turn person on side or turn head to side.
Facial Wounds
Remove any dislodged teeth or dentures that might block airway.
Use butterfly dressing to close a gaping wound (See Minor Cuts, p. 34.)
Dress with several gauze pads and four-tailed bandage, or two bandages crossed and tied at top and back of head.

*If weather is very warm and person's skin does not feel cool and clammy, covering will not be necessary.

43 Inhaled Poisons

(Including Carbon Monoxide, Carbon Dioxide, Ammonia, Chlorine, Natural Gas, Anesthetics, and other gases and fumes)

Signs & Symptoms: *different breath odor/dizziness/headache/irritability/difficulty breathing/nausea/vomiting/diarrhea/faintness/pale, bluish, or bright red lips and skin/unconsciousness*

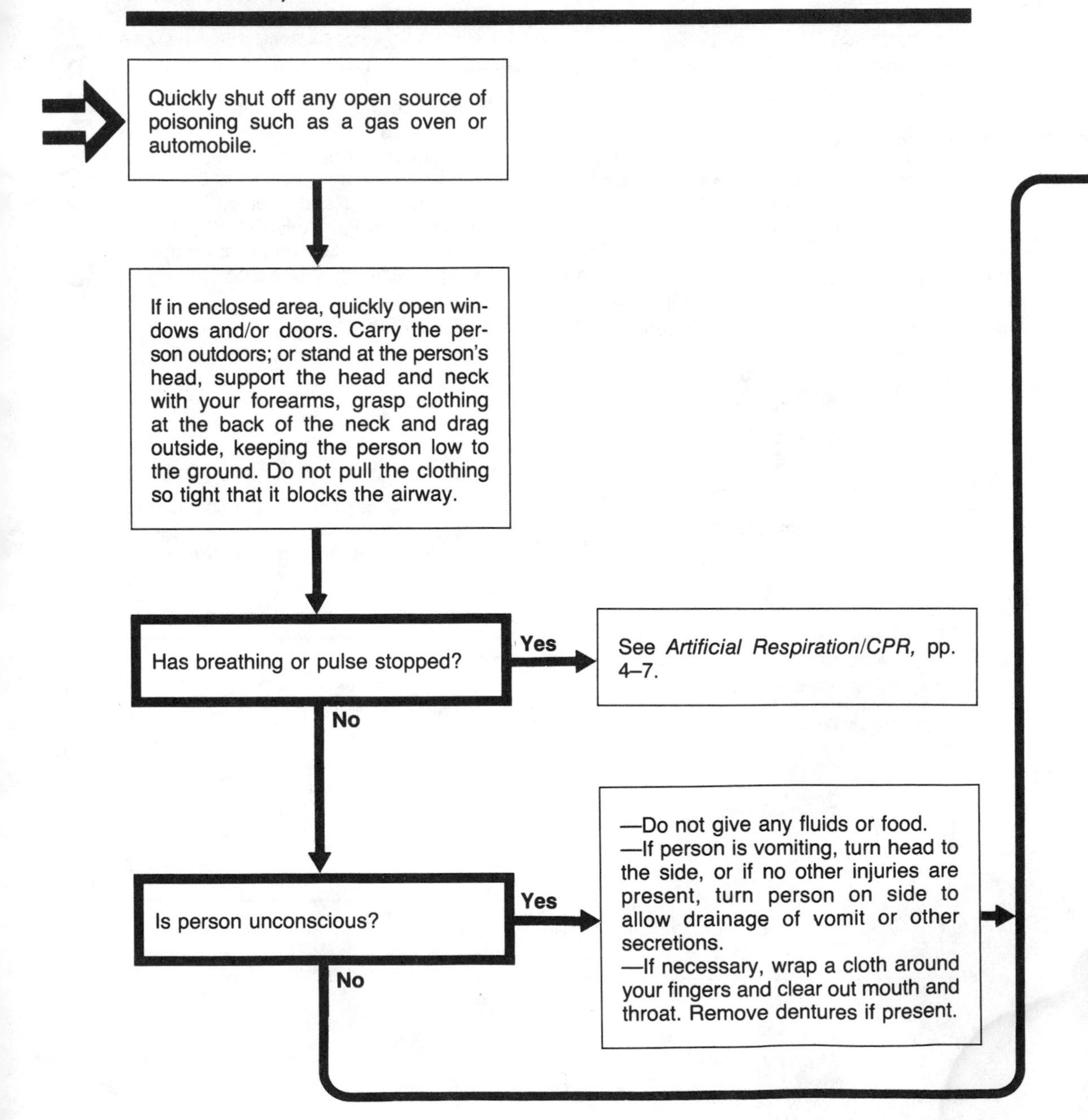

Quickly shut off any open source of poisoning such as a gas oven or automobile.
If in enclosed area, quickly open windows and/or doors. Carry the person outdoors; or stand at the person's head, support the head and neck with your forearms, grasp clothing at the back of the neck and drag outside, keeping the person low to the ground. Do not pull the clothing so tight that it blocks the airway.
Has breathing or pulse stopped?
Yes
See Artificial Respiration/CPR, pp. 4–7.
No
Is person unconscious?
Yes
—Do not give any fluids or food.
—If person is vomiting, turn head to the side, or if no other injuries are present, turn person on side to allow drainage of vomit or other secretions.
—If necessary, wrap a cloth around your fingers and clear out mouth and throat. Remove dentures if present.
No

Calm the person by talking while attending to the problem. Explain what you are doing. Try not to show anxiety; act with confidence. Your calm behavior can help to reassure the injured person.

If there are two or more rescuers, one should obtain emergency assistance and request oxygen while the other is following the procedures outlined below.

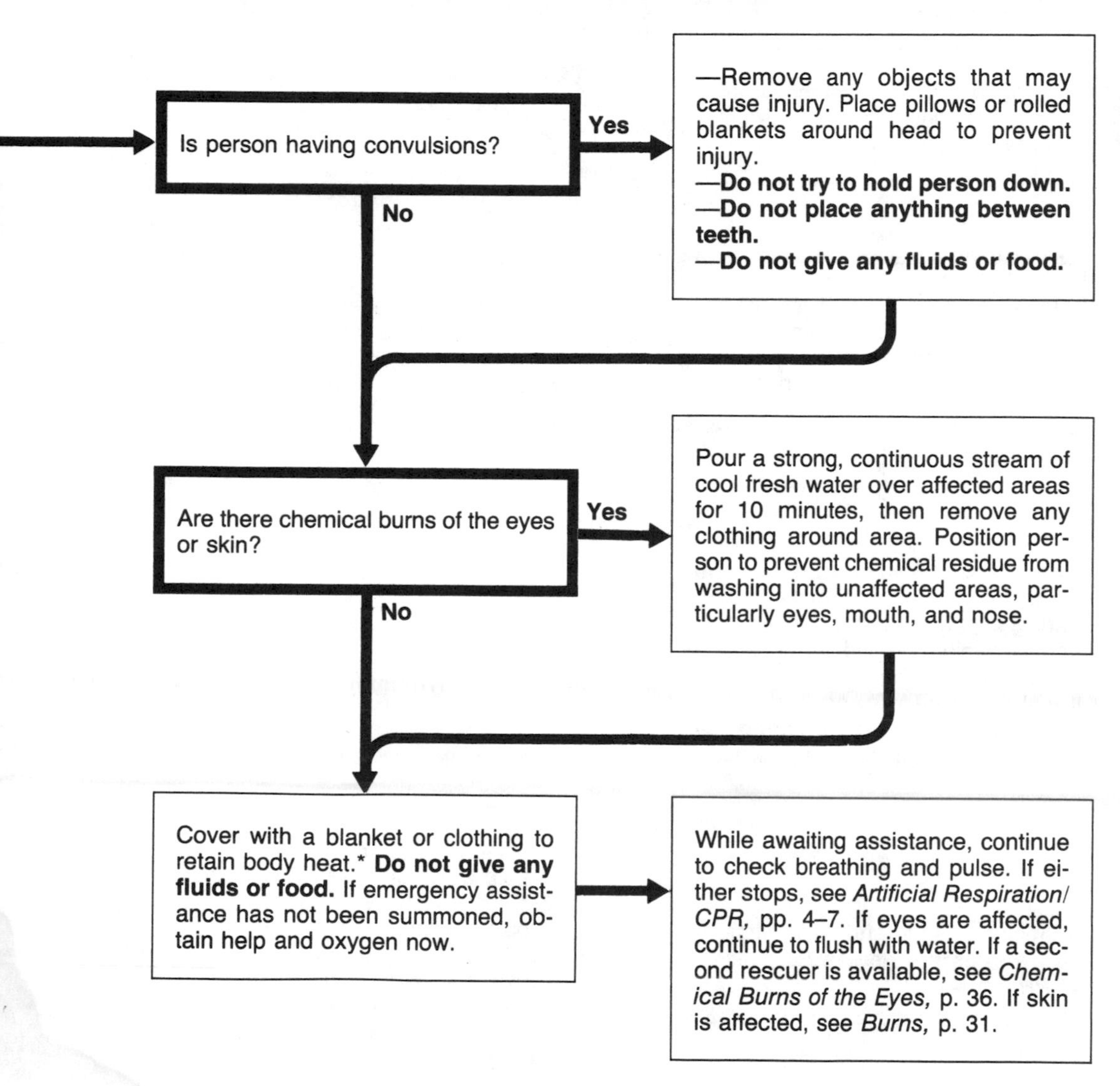
Is person having convulsions?
Yes
—Remove any objects that may cause injury. Place pillows or rolled blankets around head to prevent injury.
—Do not try to hold person down.
—Do not place anything between teeth.
—Do not give any fluids or food.
No
Are there chemical burns of the eyes or skin?
Yes
Pour a strong, continuous stream of cool fresh water over affected areas for 10 minutes, then remove any clothing around area. Position person to prevent chemical residue from washing into unaffected areas, particularly eyes, mouth, and nose.
No
Cover with a blanket or clothing to retain body heat.* Do not give any fluids or food. If emergency assistance has not been summoned, obtain help and oxygen now.
While awaiting assistance, continue to check breathing and pulse. If either stops, see Artificial Respiration/CPR, pp. 4–7. If eyes are affected, continue to flush with water. If a second rescuer is available, see Chemical Burns of the Eyes, p. 36. If skin is affected, see Burns, p. 31.

*If weather is very warm and person's skin does not feel cool and clammy, covering will not be necessary.

Insect Stings

Signs & Symptoms

Emergency allergic reaction: *breathing difficulty/faintness/cool or moist skin/swollen, red, teary eyes/hives/blotches/swollen nasal passages/nausea/vomiting/diarrhea (Very serious reactions with wheezing and collapse are apt to occur within 5–10 minutes.)*

Less serious: *local irritation or pain/moderate swelling/local redness or itching*

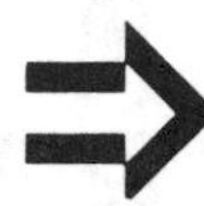

Quickly determine whether the person is experiencing a serious reaction to the insect bite.

Does person have a history of severe allergic reaction, symptoms of a severe reaction, or a severe local reaction involving head or neck?

No → If there is a stinger, remove it by scraping with a clean fingernail, tweezers, knife, or razor blade. **Do not squeeze the stinger out.**

Yes → If insect-sting kit if available, follow instructions. injecting epinephrine first. **Do not inject into limb with sting site.** If kit is not available, give antihistamine (Benadryl), or, if person has breathing difficulty, use epinephrine inhaler (Primatene Mist, etc.). **Do not give anything by mouth if person is unconscious.**

Check breathing and pulse often. If either stops, see *Artificial Respiration/CPR,* pp. 4–7.

If person was stung on an arm or leg, tie a handkerchief or cloth strip 2–5 inches above sting site. Band should be snug, but you should be able to slip a finger under it. Apply ice or cold compress above sting site. If emergency assistance has not been summoned, obtain help now.

Calm the person by talking while attending to the problem. Explain what you are doing. Try not to show anxiety; act with confidence. Your calm behavior can help to reassure the injured person.

For emergency allergic reaction, when there are two or more rescuers, one should obtain emergency assistance while the other is following the procedures outlined below.

Wash sting site with soap and water. Apply cold compresses or ice bag wrapped in towel for 15–20 minutes, then apply calamine lotion.

Watch for signs of infection or any allergic symptoms that may develop. If they appear, seek medical care.

Keep person quiet and calm. Loosen the band for 15 seconds every 10 minutes. Remove after 30 minutes. Keep sting site below heart level.

While awaiting assistance, continue to check breathing and pulse. If either stops, see *Artificial Respiration/CPR,* pp. 4–7.

45 Poison Ivy, Oak, & Sumac

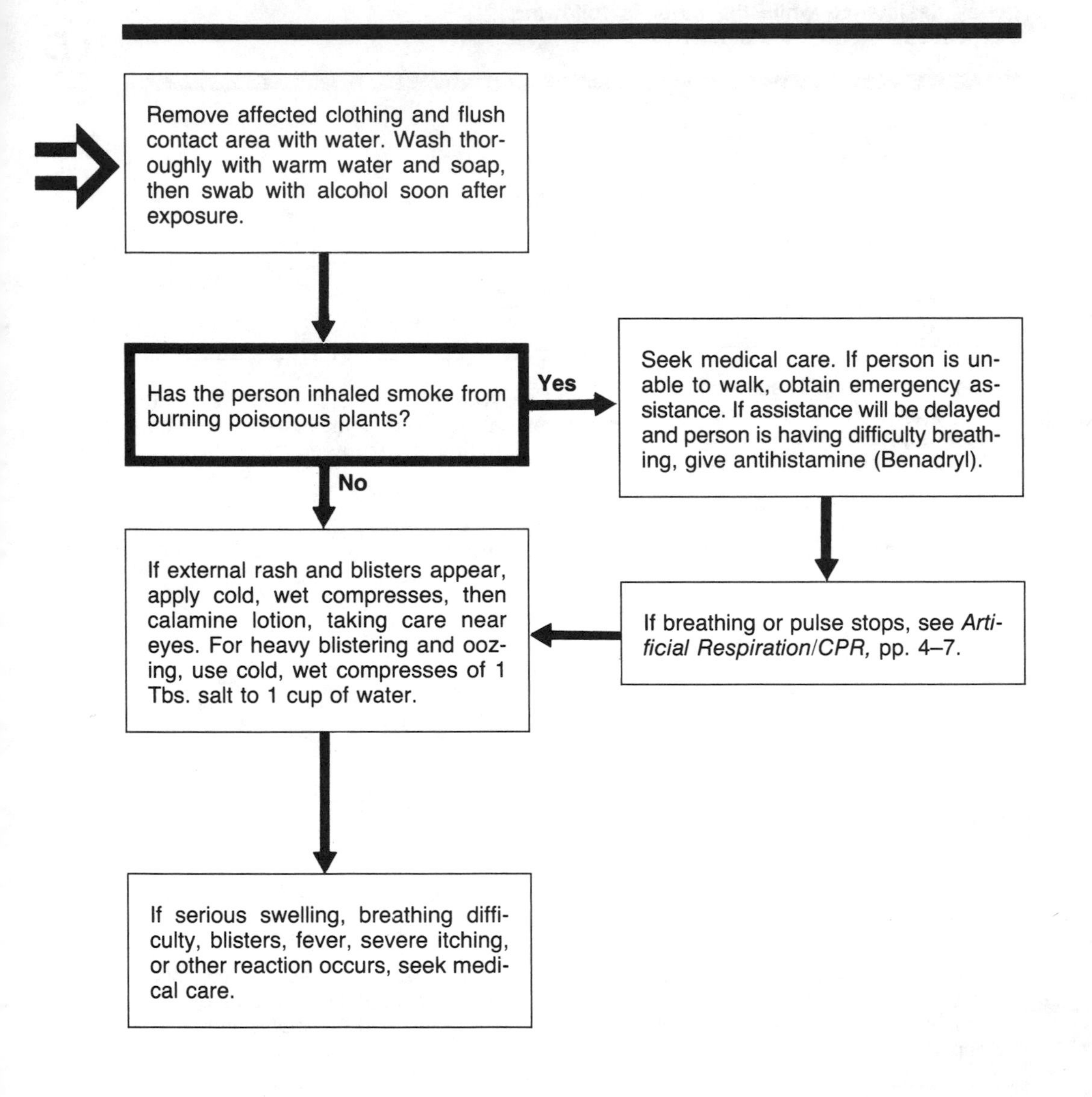

Remove affected clothing and flush contact area with water. Wash thoroughly with warm water and soap, then swab with alcohol soon after exposure.
Has the person inhaled smoke from burning poisonous plants?
Yes
Seek medical care. If person is unable to walk, obtain emergency assistance. If assistance will be delayed and person is having difficulty breathing, give antihistamine (Benadryl).
If breathing or pulse stops, see Artificial Respiration/CPR, pp. 4–7.
No
If external rash and blisters appear, apply cold, wet compresses, then calamine lotion, taking care near eyes. For heavy blistering and oozing, use cold, wet compresses of 1 Tbs. salt to 1 cup of water.
If serious swelling, breathing difficulty, blisters, fever, severe itching, or other reaction occurs, seek medical care.

Calm the person by talking while attending to the problem. Explain what you are doing. Try not to show anxiety; act with confidence. Your calm behavior can help to reassure the injured person.

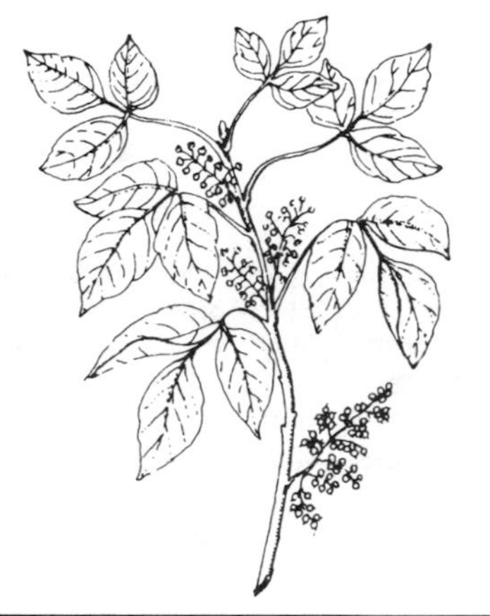

Recognize common poison plants:

Poison Ivy
Small plant, vine, or shrub common throughout U.S. except California. Shiny leaves grow in clusters of three, turning red and yellow toward fall.

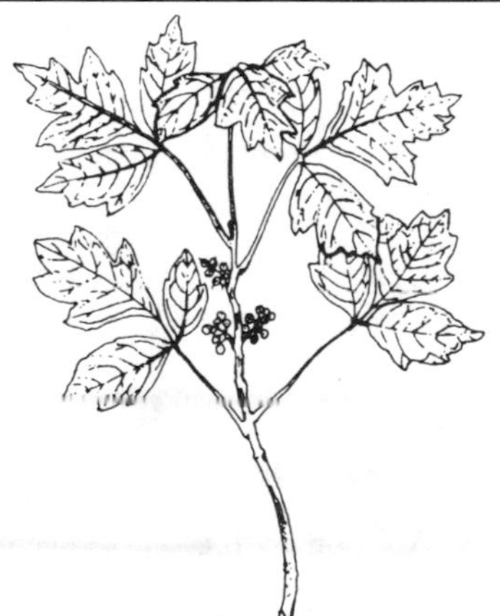

Poison Oak
Western variety grows in California and portions of adjacent states as shrub or vine closely resembling poison ivy.
More common variety grows in other areas, usually as a shrub with oluo ters of hairy, yellowish berries and undersides of leaves covered with hair.

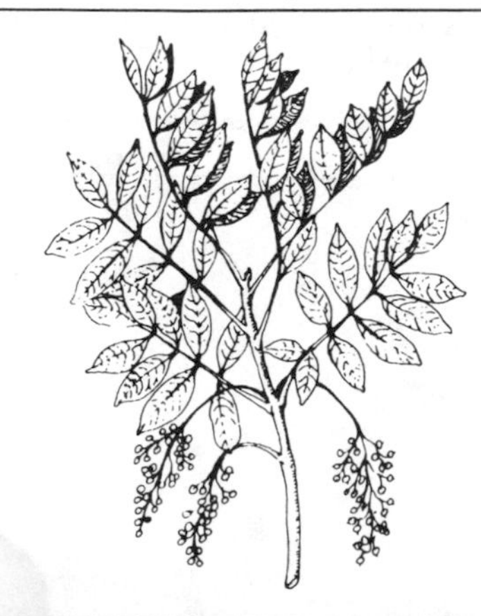

Poison Sumac
Woody shrub or small tree (5–25 feet) grows in eastern U.S., especially in moist climates.
Each leaf stalk has 7–13 leaflets with smooth edges, which turn red in fall, and cream-colored berries which hang from branches in loose clusters.

Snakebite

These procedures must be followed *immediately* after snakebite.

Signs & Symptoms:
Poisonous: *Severe reaction occurs within 30 minutes. Burning pain at bite/swelling/discoloration/weakness/dizziness/faint pulse. Coral snake reactions may appear less severe and may be delayed up to 10 hours. See maps and descriptions of poisonous snakes, next page.*

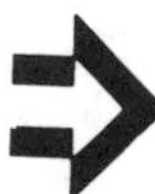

Have person lie completely quiet. Keep site of bite below heart level if possible. Remove rings, watch, bracelets.

Tie a handkerchief or cloth strip snugly around limb 2–5 inches above bite (not on joint), leaving it loose enough to slip a finger under it. (See illustration at right.) Immediately apply suction to bite without making incisions. Use suction cups in snakebite kit (directions in kit) or, if no cups are available, use mouth suction if you have no sores in mouth. Spit out venom and rinse mouth frequently (although snake venom is not a stomach poison). Apply suction for 15 minutes.

After 15 minutes, is there pain, swelling, numbness, discoloration around the bite?

No

Wash skin around wound with soap and water. If emergency assistance has not been summoned, obtain help now.

Yes

—If swelling begins to extend above the band, apply second band above new swelling; leave first band in place.
—Wash skin around wound with soap and water.

Obtain emergency assistance if not already summoned.

Will person receive medical assistance within 60 minutes of snakebite?
OR
Was the person bitten by coral snake?

No

Yes

Calm the person by talking while attending to the problem. Explain what you are doing. Try not to show anxiety; act with confidence. Your calm behavior can help to reassure the injured person.

If there are two or more rescuers, one should obtain emergency assistance while the other is following the procedures outlined below.

—Sterilize knife or razor blade with alcohol or by holding in a flame.
—Make a linear, *not crosswise,* incision through each fang mark, about ⅛ to ¼ inch long, not more than ⅛ inch deep. **Do not** cut deeply enough to damage nerves or muscles. **Do not** cut through a vein. (*See illustration below.*)

—Apply suction with cups in snakebite kit. (Directions in kit.) If not enough cups to cover all incisions, rotate them every 3–5 minutes. If no cups are available, use mouth suction if you have no open sores in mouth. Spit out venom and rinse mouth frequently (although snake venom is not a stomach poison).

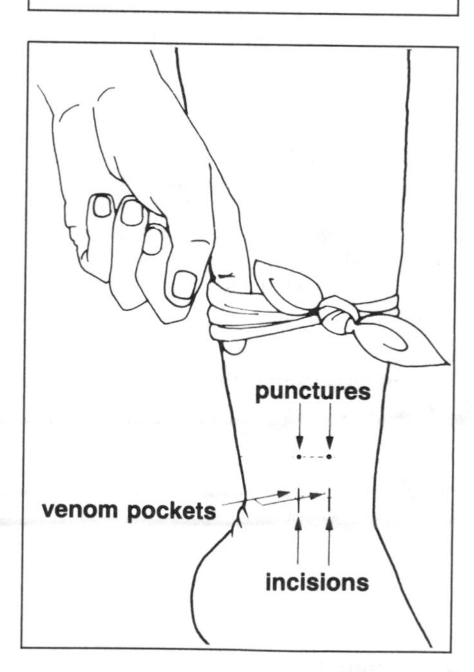
punctures
venom pockets
incisions

If snakebite kit is available, use antivenin as directed in package. Be sure to test for allergy as instructed.

While awaiting assistance, watch breathing and pulse. If either stops, see *Artificial Respiration/CPR,* pp. 4–7.

Wash bite again with soap and water, then bandage. Cover with blanket to retain body heat.* Continue to check breathing.

*If weather is very warm and person's skin does not feel cool and clammy, covering will not be necessary.

46A Recognize common poisonous snakes

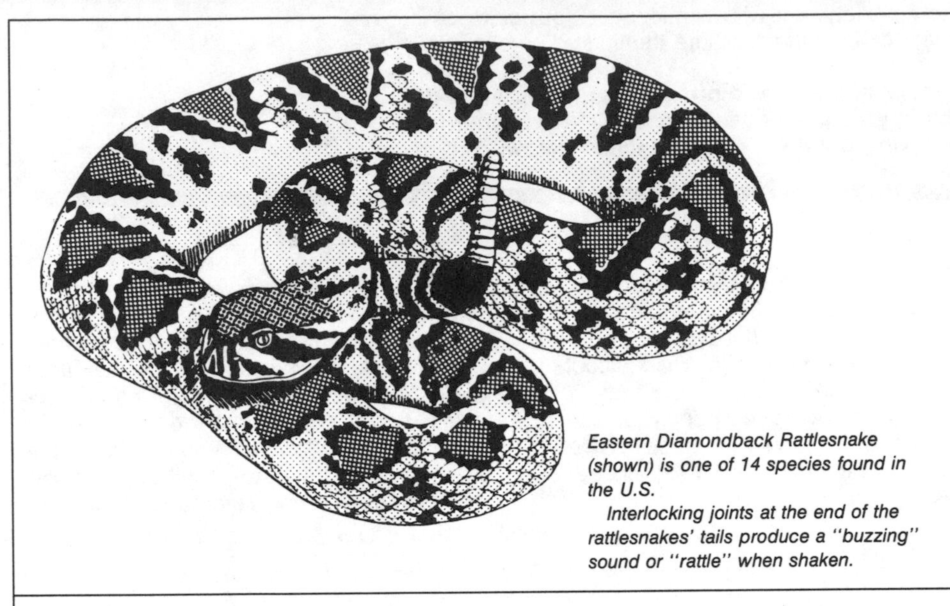

Eastern Diamondback Rattlesnake (shown) is one of 14 species found in the U.S.

Interlocking joints at the end of the rattlesnakes' tails produce a "buzzing" sound or "rattle" when shaken.

Eastern Diamondback Rattlesnake

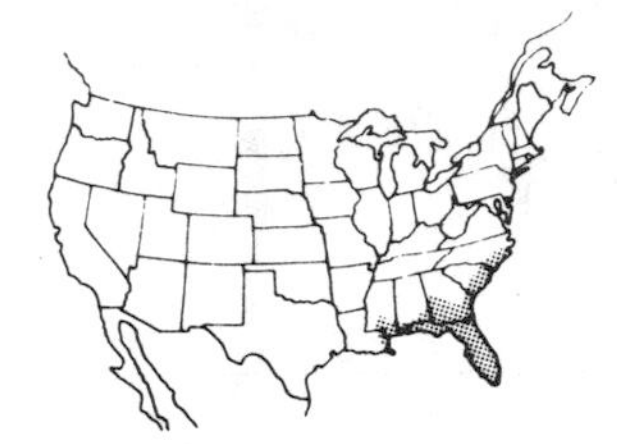

Description Dark diamonds with light borders along a tan or light brown background. Diamonds gradually changing to bands in tail. Diagonal brown lines on the sides of face, vertical on snout.
Habitat Lowland thickets, palmettos, flatwoods.

Canebrake and Timber Rattlesnake

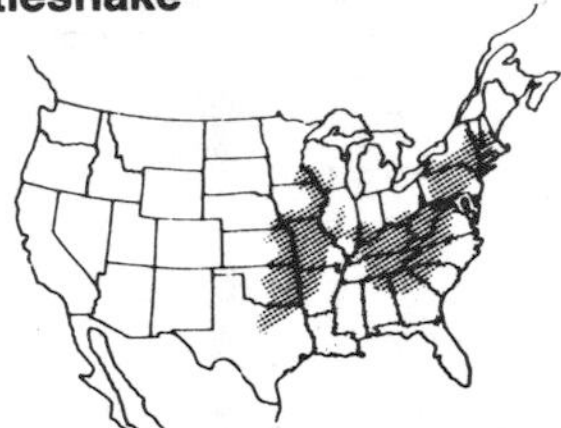

Description South: Dark streak from canebrake snake's eye to mouth; dark chevrons and rusty stripe along midline. Pink to tan ground color darker toward tail, which is black in adults. North: timber rattlesnake has yellowish ground color and a dark phase in part of its range.
Habitat Canebrake: lowland brush, and stream borders. Timber rattlesnake: rocky wooded hills.

Western Diamondback Rattlesnake

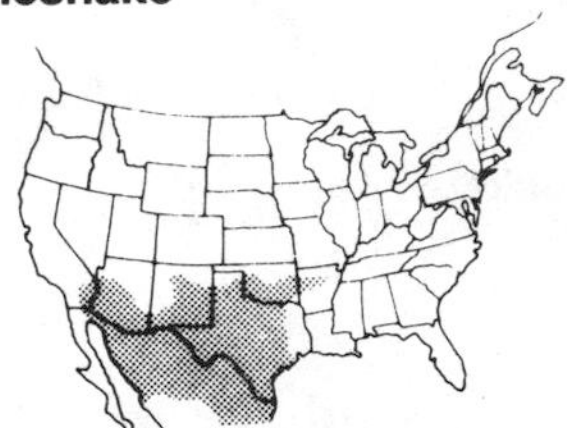

Description Light brown to black diamond-shaped blotches along light gray, tan, and, in some localities, pink background. Black and white bands of about equal width around tail and black basal rattle.
Habitat Diverse terrain: dry, sparsely wooded, rocky hills, flat desert and coastal sand dunes. Often found in agricultural land and near towns.

Copperhead

Northern Copperhead (shown here) and other Copperheads in the U.S. vibrate their tails rapidly when alarmed.

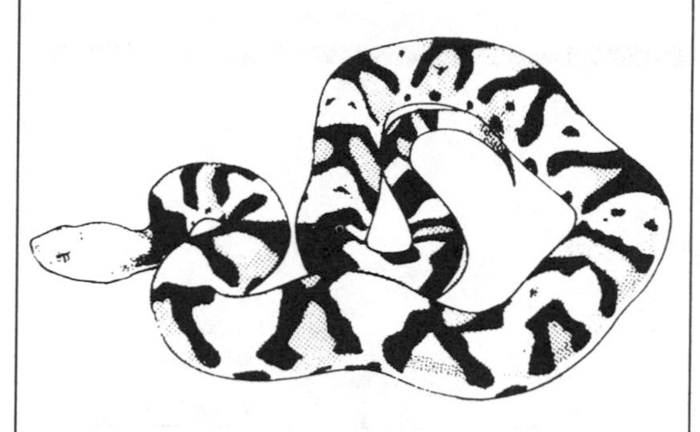

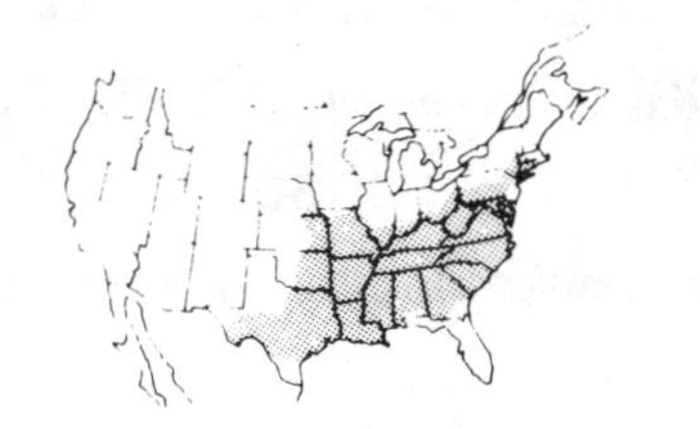

Description Large chestnut brown cross bands on a pale pinkish or reddish-brown surface; and coppery tinge of head.
Habitat North: wooded mountains; hills; wild, damp meadows; along stone walls; in slab or sawdust piles. South: lowland swamps and uplands; sometimes found in wooded suburbs.

Coral Snakes

Eastern Coral (below) and Texas Coral are dangerously poisonous although their small mouths and short fangs make it difficult to bite most parts of the body.

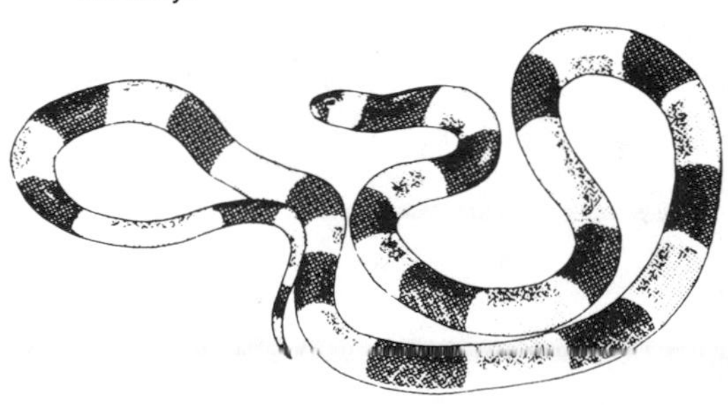

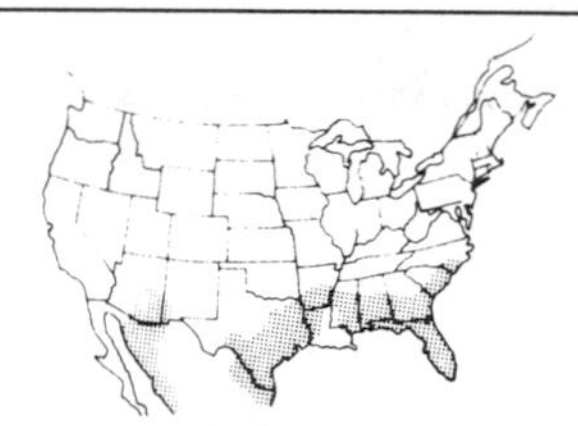

Description Red and black rings, wider than the interspaced yellow rings. Black snout, round pupils; no facial pits.
Habitat East: grassland; dry, open woods; and frequently suburban areas. West: (much less dangerous), desert and semidesert where there is loose soil and rocks.

Cottonmouth (water moccasin)

Eastern Cottonmouth (below). Florida and Western Cottonmouths, are frequently confused with several non-poisonous water snakes.

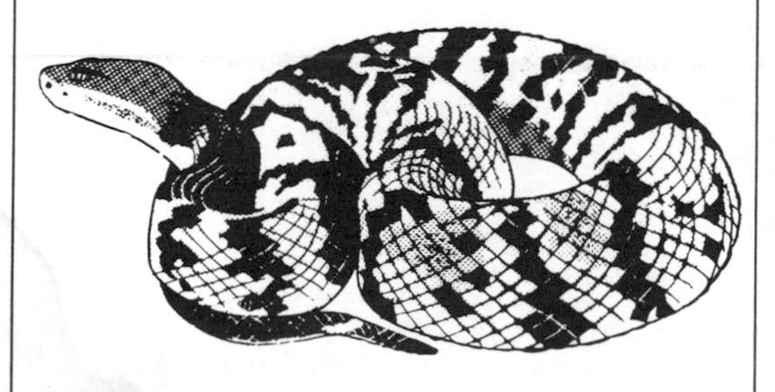

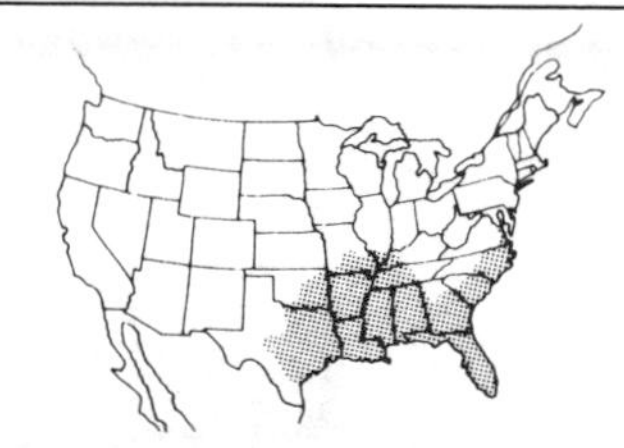

Description Dark blotches on brown or olive body. Heavy body and broad flat head.
Habitat Semiaquatic.

Spider or Scorpion Bites

Black Widow, Tarantula Brown Recluse, Scorpion

Signs & Symptoms: *rigid abdominal muscles without tenderness/breathing difficulty/slurred speech/restlessness/muscle cramps/nausea, vomiting/blister at site/many other possible signs & symptoms (see next page).*

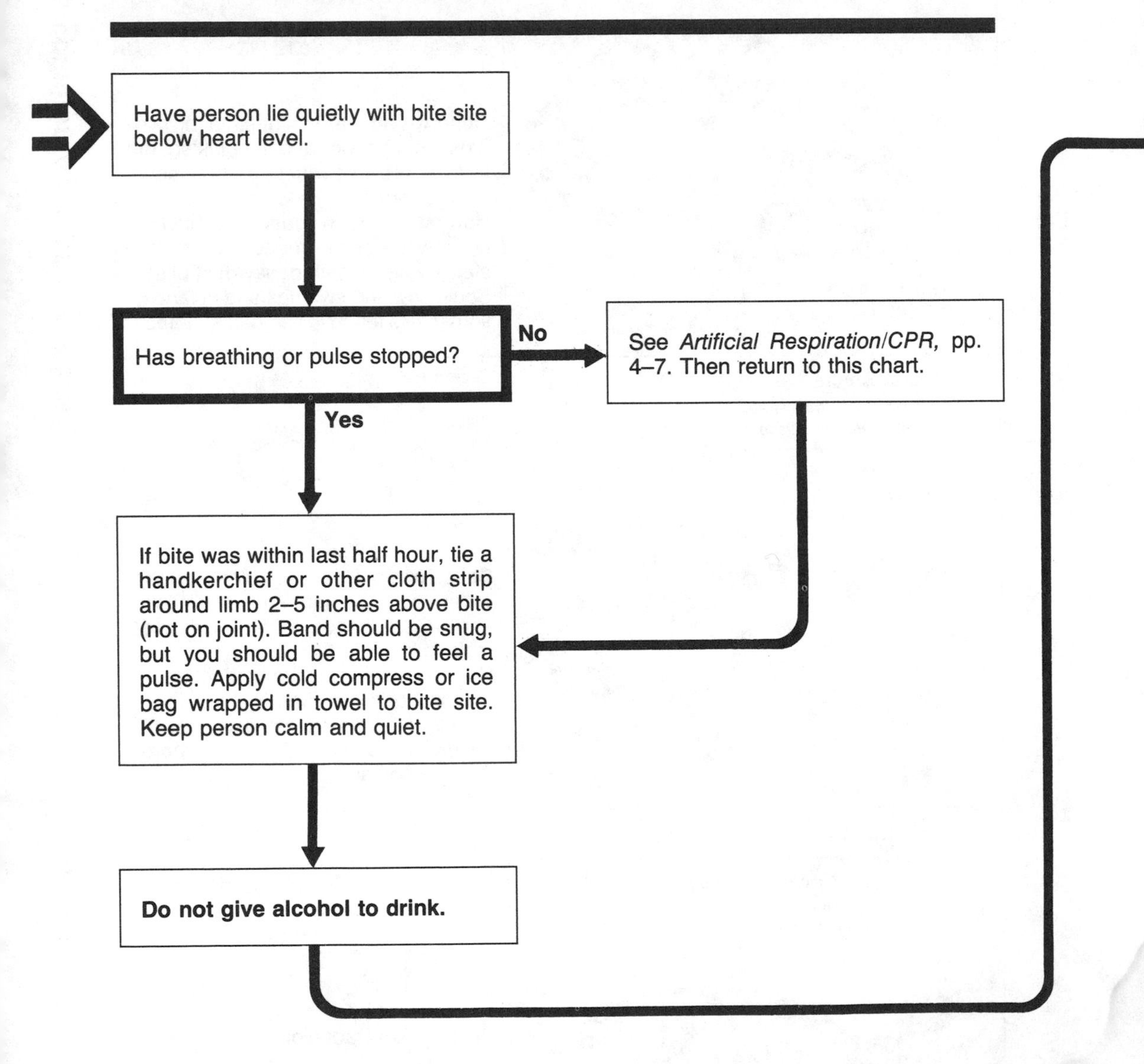

Have person lie quietly with bite site below heart level.
Has breathing or pulse stopped?
No
See *Artificial Respiration/CPR,* pp. 4–7. Then return to this chart.
Yes
If bite was within last half hour, tie a handkerchief or other cloth strip around limb 2–5 inches above bite (not on joint). Band should be snug, but you should be able to feel a pulse. Apply cold compress or ice bag wrapped in towel to bite site. Keep person calm and quiet.
Do not give alcohol to drink.

Calm the person by talking while attending to the problem. Explain what you are doing. Try not to show anxiety; act with confidence. Your calm behavior can help to reassure the injured person.

If there are two or more rescuers, one should obtain emergency assistance while the other is following the procedures outlined below.

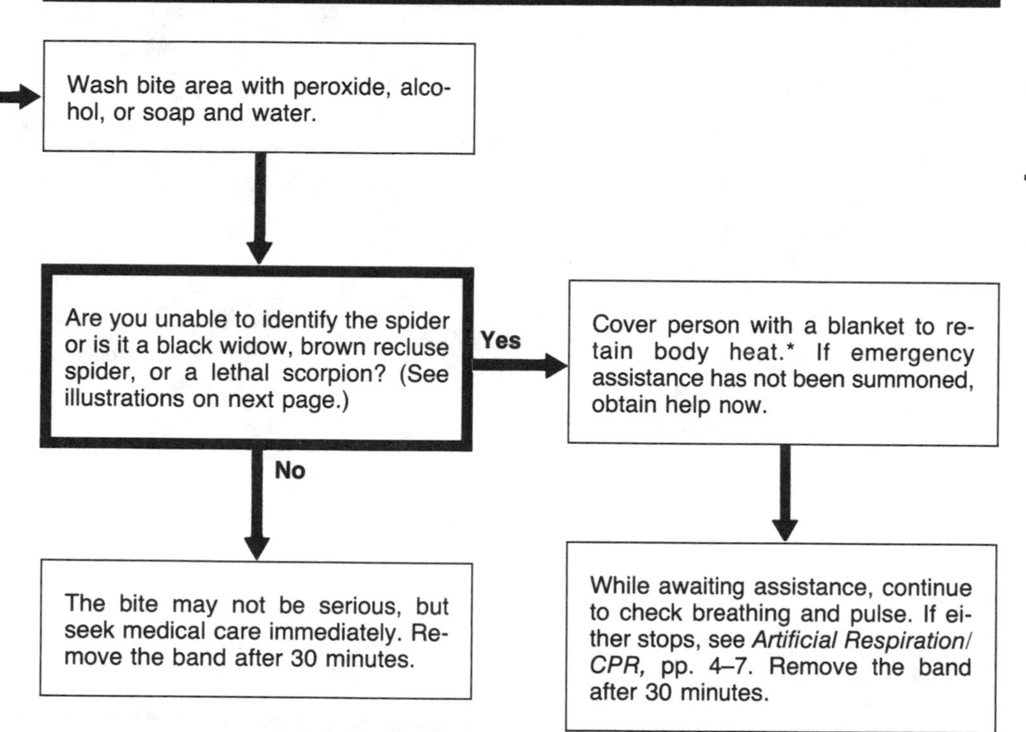
Wash bite area with peroxide, alcohol, or soap and water.
Are you unable to identify the spider or is it a black widow, brown recluse spider, or a lethal scorpion? (See illustrations on next page.)
Yes
Cover person with a blanket to retain body heat.* If emergency assistance has not been summoned, obtain help now.
While awaiting assistance, continue to check breathing and pulse. If either stops, see *Artificial Respiration/CPR,* pp. 4–7. Remove the band after 30 minutes.
No
The bite may not be serious, but seek medical care immediately. Remove the band after 30 minutes.

*If weather is very warm and person's skin does not feel cool and clammy, covering will not be necessary.

47A Recognize poisonous spiders

Black Widow Spider

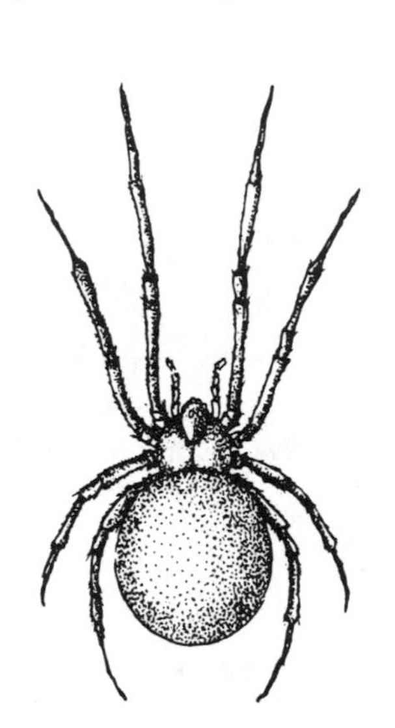

Coal-black, bulbous spider ¾–1½ in. long. Bright red hourglass on abdomen. (Be especially cautious in outdoor toilets, where these spiders inhabit underside of seats.)

Possible Signs & Symptoms

- sensation of pinprick or minor burning at time of bite
- appearance of small punctures (but sometimes none)
- within 15–60 minutes, intense pain at site spreading quickly
- profuse sweating
- rigid abdominal muscles without abdominal tenderness
- other muscle spasms
- breathing difficulty
- slurred speech, poor coordination
- dilated pupils
- generalized swelling of face and extremities

Tarantula

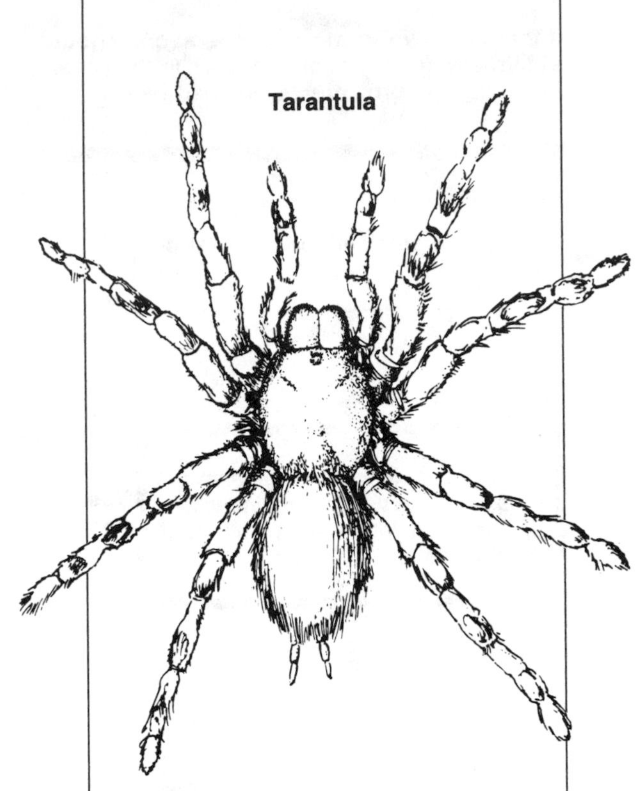

Large, hairy spiders . . . dark brown to black. Up to 7 in. long.

Possible Signs & Symptoms

- may be similar to Black Widow Spider; however, tarantula bites are generally no worse than a bee sting.

Brown Recluse Spider

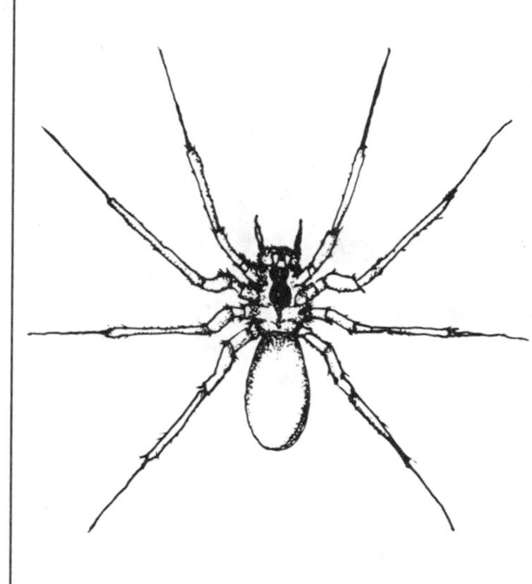

Brownish, rather flat, ½–⅝ in. long. Dark brown "violin" on underside. Usually found in clothes closets and dark locations in buildings.

Possible Signs & Symptoms
- blister at site
- generalized rash
- joint pain
- chills
- fever
- nausea & vomiting
- pain may become severe after 8 hours

Scorpion

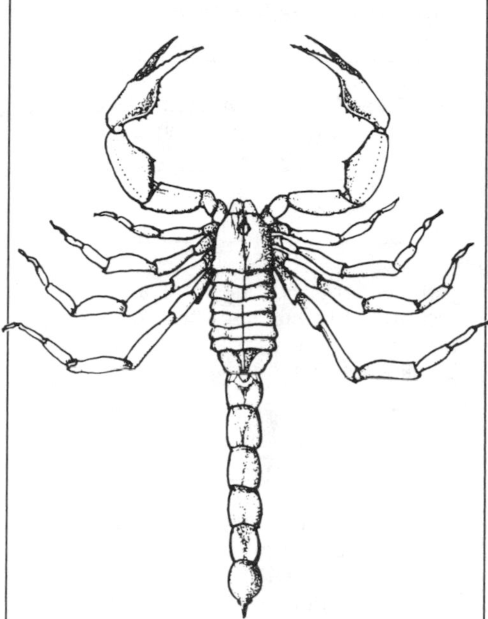

¾–3 in. long. Yellow to greenish-yellow. Lethal variety found only in Arizona and Southern California. Night animal. Hides in dark places, such as shoes and boots.

Possible Signs & Symptoms
- prickling sensation at time of bite, quickly followed by severe pain
- site becomes extremely sensitive
- restlessness
- severe breathing difficulty
- convulsion
- muscle cramps, nausea, vomiting
- high fever
- headache, dizziness
- abdominal pain
- profuse sweating

Sprain or Strain

Signs & Symptoms:
Sprain (joint): *swelling and discoloration of joint area/pain with movement/no deformity of the joint*
Strain (muscle, ligament, or tendon): *sharp, tearing pain/possible muscle spasm/possible discoloration (later)/gradual stiffening of area*

If you suspect *Fractures,* see p. 41.

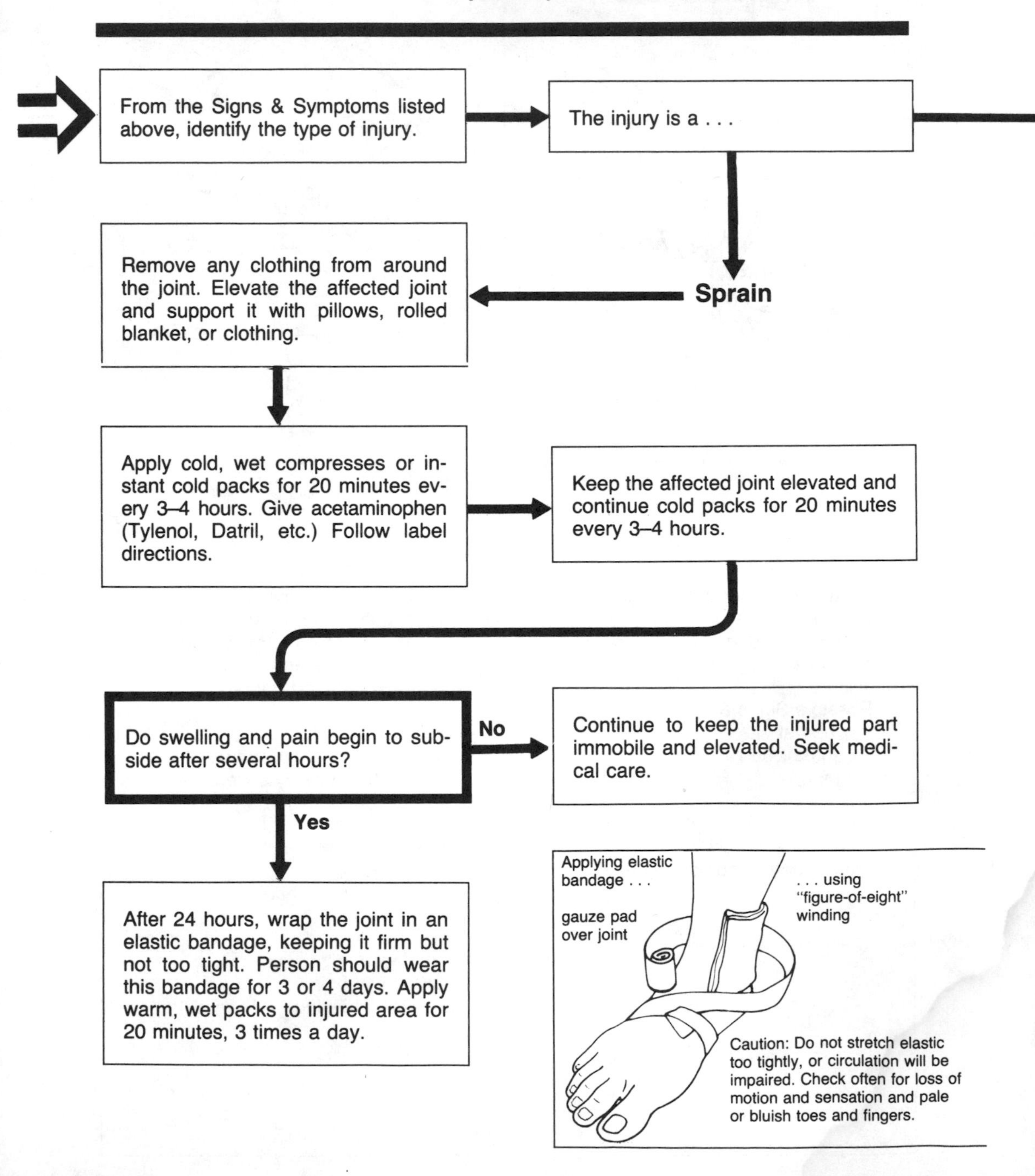
From the Signs & Symptoms listed above, identify the type of injury.
The injury is a . . .
Sprain
Remove any clothing from around the joint. Elevate the affected joint and support it with pillows, rolled blanket, or clothing.
Apply cold, wet compresses or instant cold packs for 20 minutes every 3–4 hours. Give acetaminophen (Tylenol, Datril, etc.) Follow label directions.
Keep the affected joint elevated and continue cold packs for 20 minutes every 3–4 hours.
Do swelling and pain begin to subside after several hours?
No
Continue to keep the injured part immobile and elevated. Seek medical care.
Yes
After 24 hours, wrap the joint in an elastic bandage, keeping it firm but not too tight. Person should wear this bandage for 3 or 4 days. Apply warm, wet packs to injured area for 20 minutes, 3 times a day.
Applying elastic bandage . . .
gauze pad over joint
. . . using "figure-of-eight" winding
Caution: Do not stretch elastic too tightly, or circulation will be impaired. Check often for loss of motion and sensation and pale or bluish toes and fingers.

Calm the person by talking while attending to the problem. Explain what you are doing. Try not to show anxiety; act with confidence. Your calm behavior can help to reassure the injured person.

If injury was the result of a vehicular or job-related accident, the person should be examined by a physician for possible additional injuries or complications.

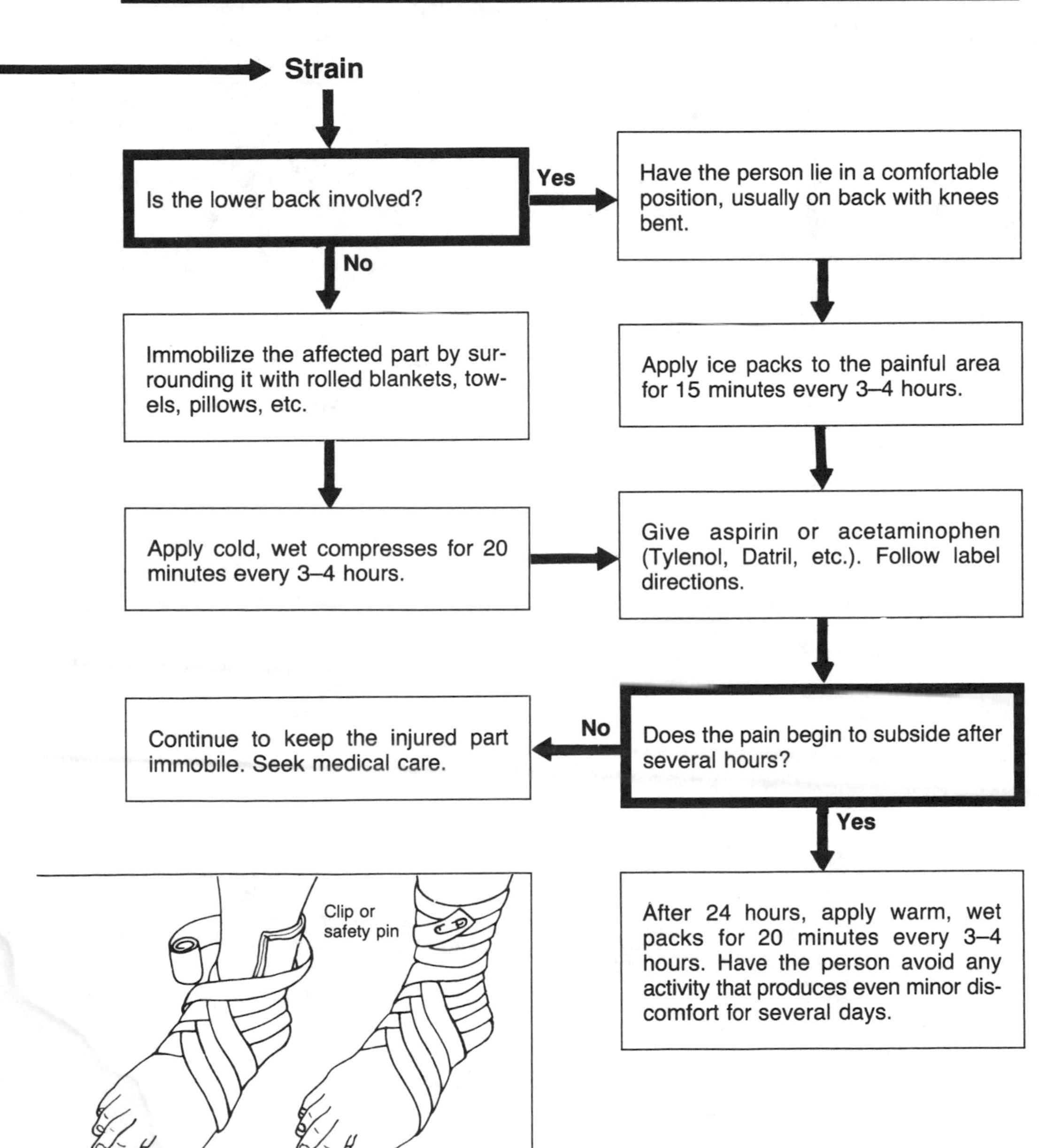
Strain
Is the lower back involved?
Yes
Have the person lie in a comfortable position, usually on back with knees bent.
Apply ice packs to the painful area for 15 minutes every 3–4 hours.
No
Immobilize the affected part by surrounding it with rolled blankets, towels, pillows, etc.
Apply cold, wet compresses for 20 minutes every 3–4 hours.
Give aspirin or acetaminophen (Tylenol, Datril, etc.). Follow label directions.
Does the pain begin to subside after several hours?
No
Continue to keep the injured part immobile. Seek medical care.
Yes
After 24 hours, apply warm, wet packs for 20 minutes every 3–4 hours. Have the person avoid any activity that produces even minor discomfort for several days.
Clip or safety pin

49 Tick Removal

Check for ticks on exposed areas of the body. (Don't forget to check the head and behind the ears.)

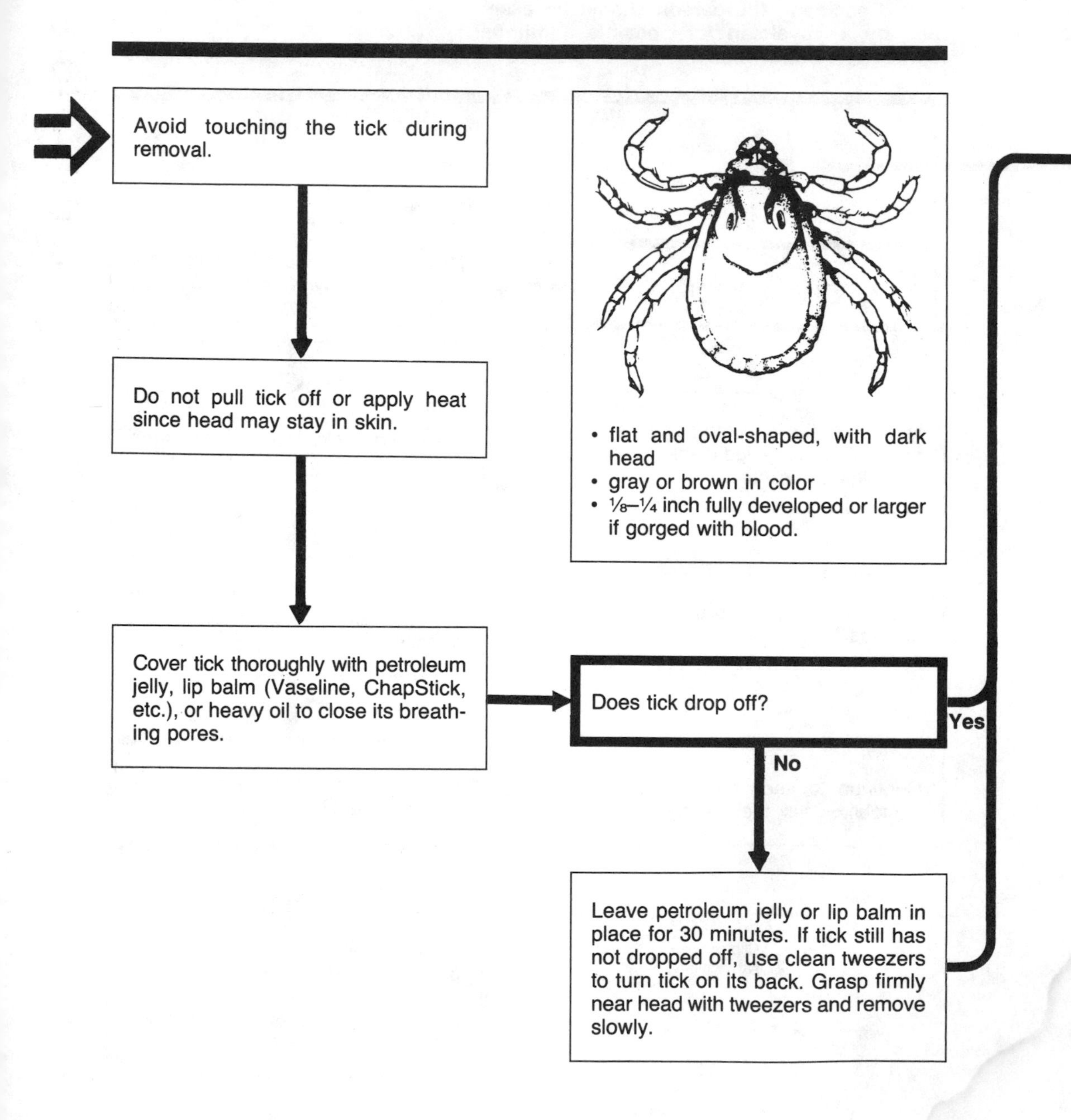

Avoid touching the tick during removal.
Do not pull tick off or apply heat since head may stay in skin.
Cover tick thoroughly with petroleum jelly, lip balm (Vaseline, ChapStick, etc.), or heavy oil to close its breathing pores.
• flat and oval-shaped, with dark head
• gray or brown in color
• ⅛–¼ inch fully developed or larger if gorged with blood.
Does tick drop off?
Yes
No
Leave petroleum jelly or lip balm in place for 30 minutes. If tick still has not dropped off, use clean tweezers to turn tick on its back. Grasp firmly near head with tweezers and remove slowly.

Calm the person by talking while attending to the problem. Explain what you are doing. Try not to show anxiety; act with confidence. Your calm behavior can help to reassure the injured person.

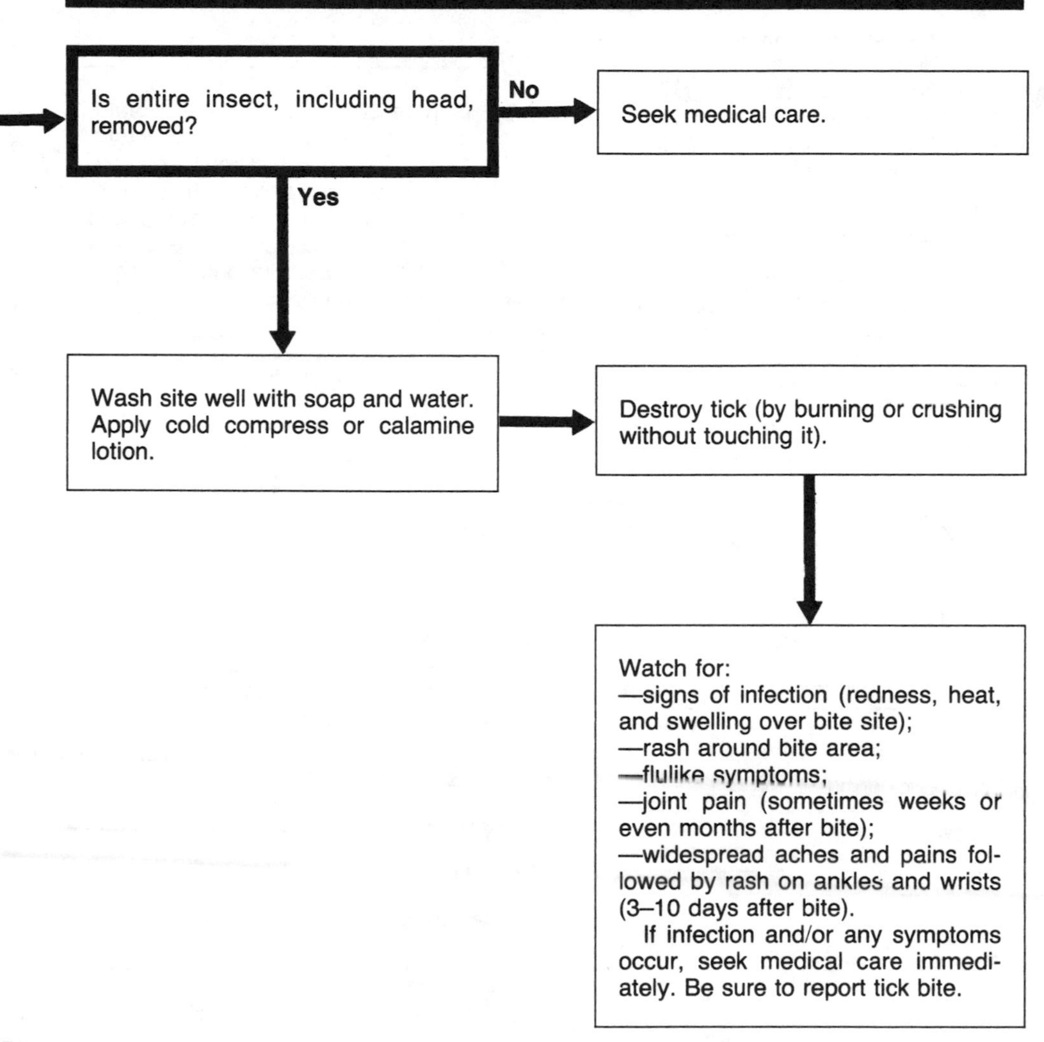
Is entire insect, including head, removed?
No
Seek medical care.
Yes
Wash site well with soap and water. Apply cold compress or calamine lotion.
Destroy tick (by burning or crushing without touching it).
Watch for:
—signs of infection (redness, heat, and swelling over bite site);
—rash around bite area;
—flulike symptoms;
—joint pain (sometimes weeks or even months after bite);
—widespread aches and pains followed by rash on ankles and wrists (3–10 days after bite).
If infection and/or any symptoms occur, seek medical care immediately. Be sure to report tick bite.

50 Deep Wound

Definition: *heavy bleeding/involvement of underlying tissues, including muscles, nerves, tendons, or major blood vessels.*

If there are two or more rescuers, one should obtain emergency assistance while the other is following the procedures outlined below.

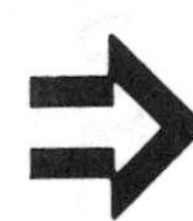

Have the person sit or lie in a comfortable position. Immobilize the injured part, if necessary, with pillows or rolled blankets; then elevate it to help reduce bleeding. Cut clothing away from wound.

If there is a gaping facial wound, use butterfly dressing to close it (see *Minor Cuts*, p. 34). Dress with several gauze pads and four-tailed bandage or two bandages crossed and tied at top and back of head. (Be careful not to choke person.) Then see Box A on opposite page.

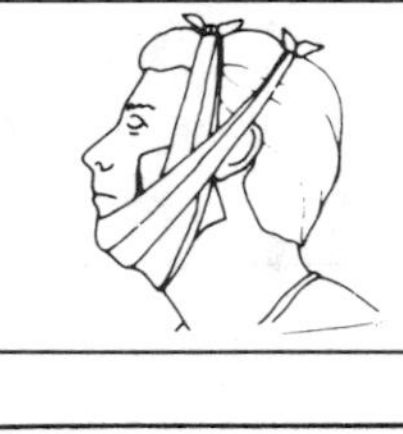

For other wounds, cover with a thick, sterile gauze pad (or other clean material) and apply gentle, firm, continuous, direct pressure with the palm of your hand.

Do not remove the original pad; let blood soak through and begin to clot. If necessary, place additional pads over the original and continue to apply pressure for 5-10 minutes.

Does the bleeding slow down?

Yes

No

Apply pressure with fingers and thumb to the major artery supplying blood to the wounded area (shown below).

Pressure Points

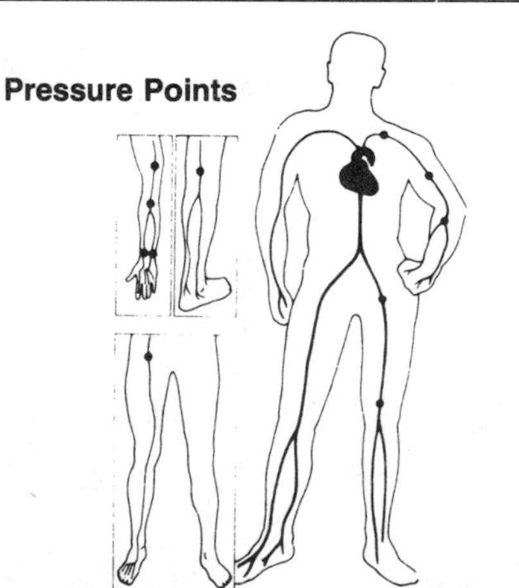

Does bleeding stop or slow down considerably?

Yes

No

Wrap a strip of cloth or other bandage over pad(s). Pull firmly to apply some pressure without cutting off blood circulation. Check position of fingers and thumb and reapply pressure to artery.

Calm the person by talking while attending to the problem. Explain what you are doing. Try not to show anxiety; act with confidence. Your calm behavior can help to reassure the injured person.

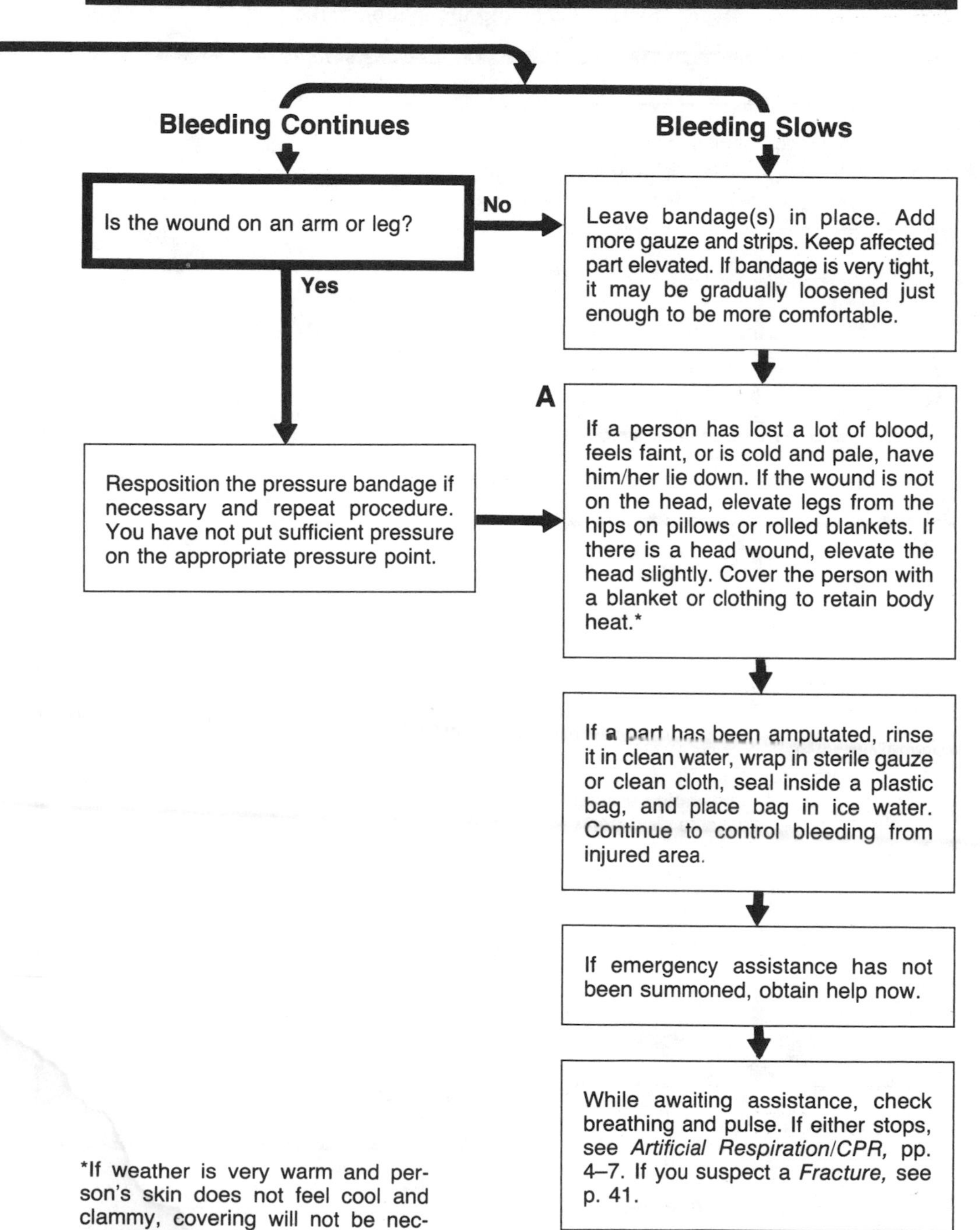
Bleeding Continues
Bleeding Slows
Is the wound on an arm or leg?
No
Yes
Leave bandage(s) in place. Add more gauze and strips. Keep affected part elevated. If bandage is very tight, it may be gradually loosened just enough to be more comfortable.
A
If a person has lost a lot of blood, feels faint, or is cold and pale, have him/her lie down. If the wound is not on the head, elevate legs from the hips on pillows or rolled blankets. If there is a head wound, elevate the head slightly. Cover the person with a blanket or clothing to retain body heat.*
Resposition the pressure bandage if necessary and repeat procedure. You have not put sufficient pressure on the appropriate pressure point.
If a part has been amputated, rinse it in clean water, wrap in sterile gauze or clean cloth, seal inside a plastic bag, and place bag in ice water. Continue to control bleeding from injured area.
If emergency assistance has not been summoned, obtain help now.
While awaiting assistance, check breathing and pulse. If either stops, see Artificial Respiration/CPR, pp. 4–7. If you suspect a Fracture, see p. 41.

*If weather is very warm and person's skin does not feel cool and clammy, covering will not be necessary.

Cold Exposure

Signs & Symptoms: *low body temperature/ uncontrollable shivering/poor muscle coordination/ shallow breathing/mental confusion/drowsiness/ numbness/possible loss of consciousness*

If there is more than one rescuer, one should obtain emergency assistance while the other is aiding the injured person.

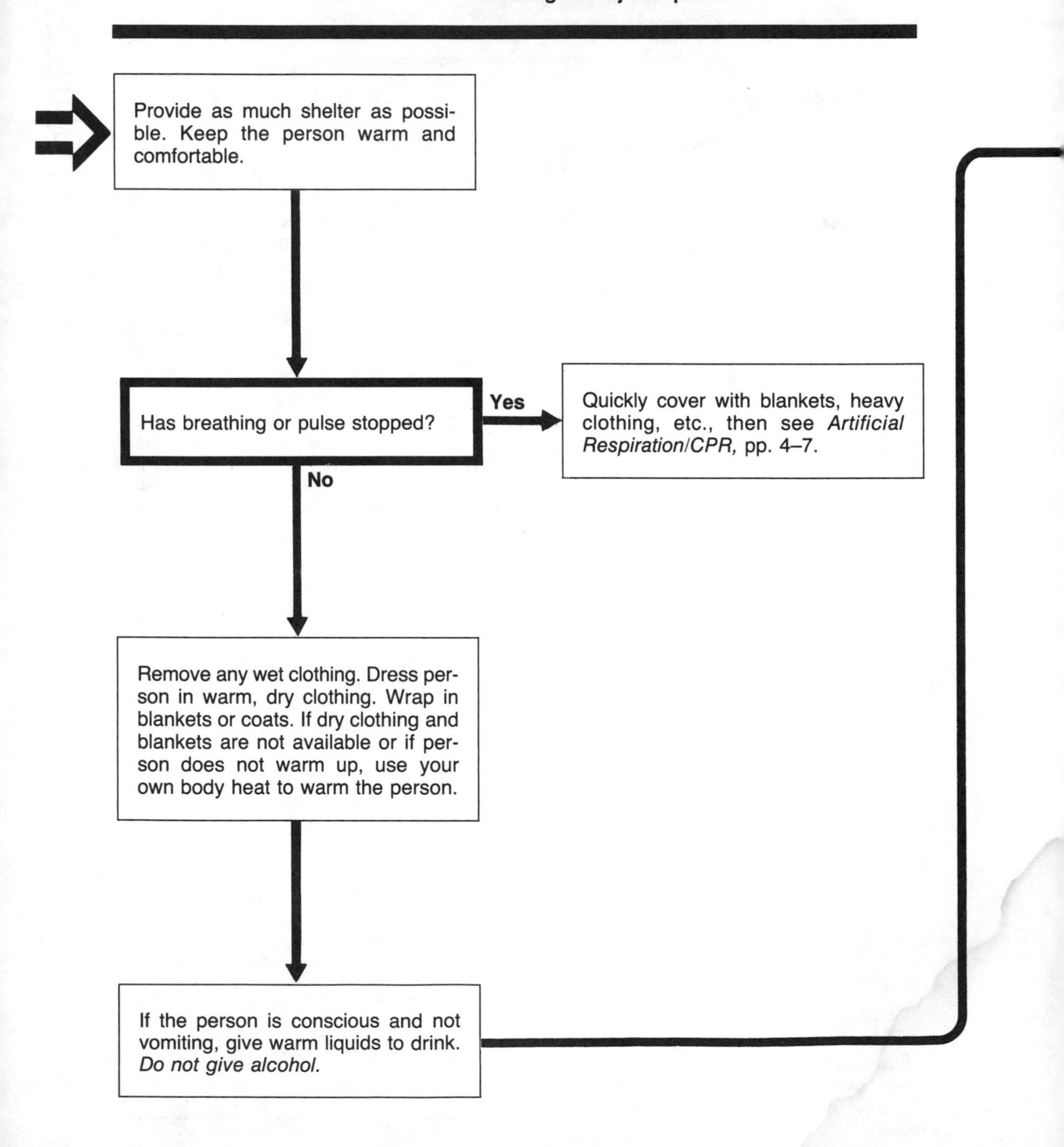

Provide as much shelter as possible. Keep the person warm and comfortable.
Has breathing or pulse stopped?
Yes
Quickly cover with blankets, heavy clothing, etc., then see Artificial Respiration/CPR, pp. 4–7.
No
Remove any wet clothing. Dress person in warm, dry clothing. Wrap in blankets or coats. If dry clothing and blankets are not available or if person does not warm up, use your own body heat to warm the person.
If the person is conscious and not vomiting, give warm liquids to drink. Do not give alcohol.

Calm the person by talking while attending to the problem. Explain what you are doing. Try not to show anxiety; act with confidence. Your calm behavior can help to reassure the injured person.

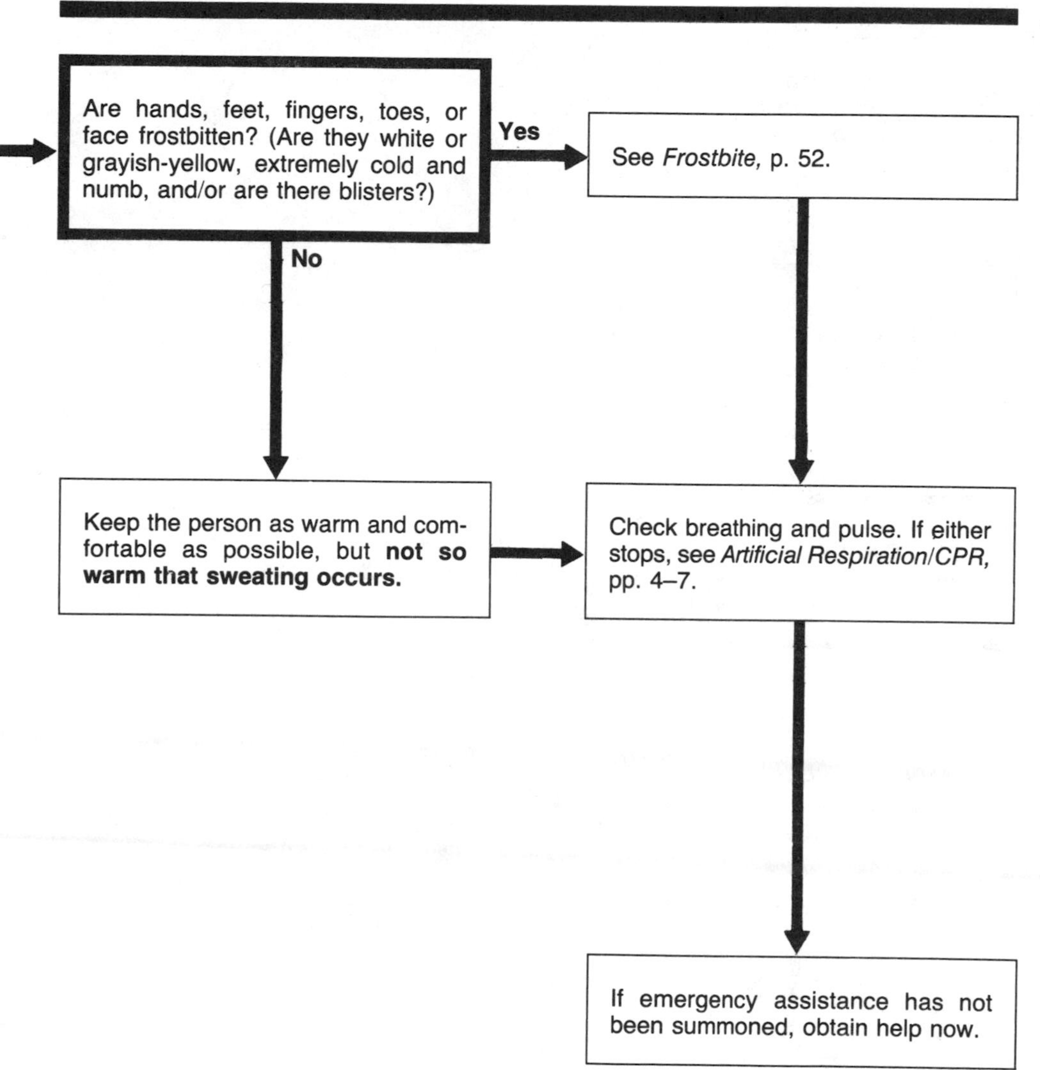
Are hands, feet, fingers, toes, or face frostbitten? (Are they white or grayish-yellow, extremely cold and numb, and/or are there blisters?)
Yes
See *Frostbite,* p. 52.
No
Keep the person as warm and comfortable as possible, but **not so warm that sweating occurs.**
Check breathing and pulse. If either stops, see *Artificial Respiration/CPR,* pp. 4–7.
If emergency assistance has not been summoned, obtain help now.

Frostbite

Signs & Symptoms: *possible pain in early stage/ skin white or grayish-yellow/extreme coldness and numbness of affected part/possible blisters.*

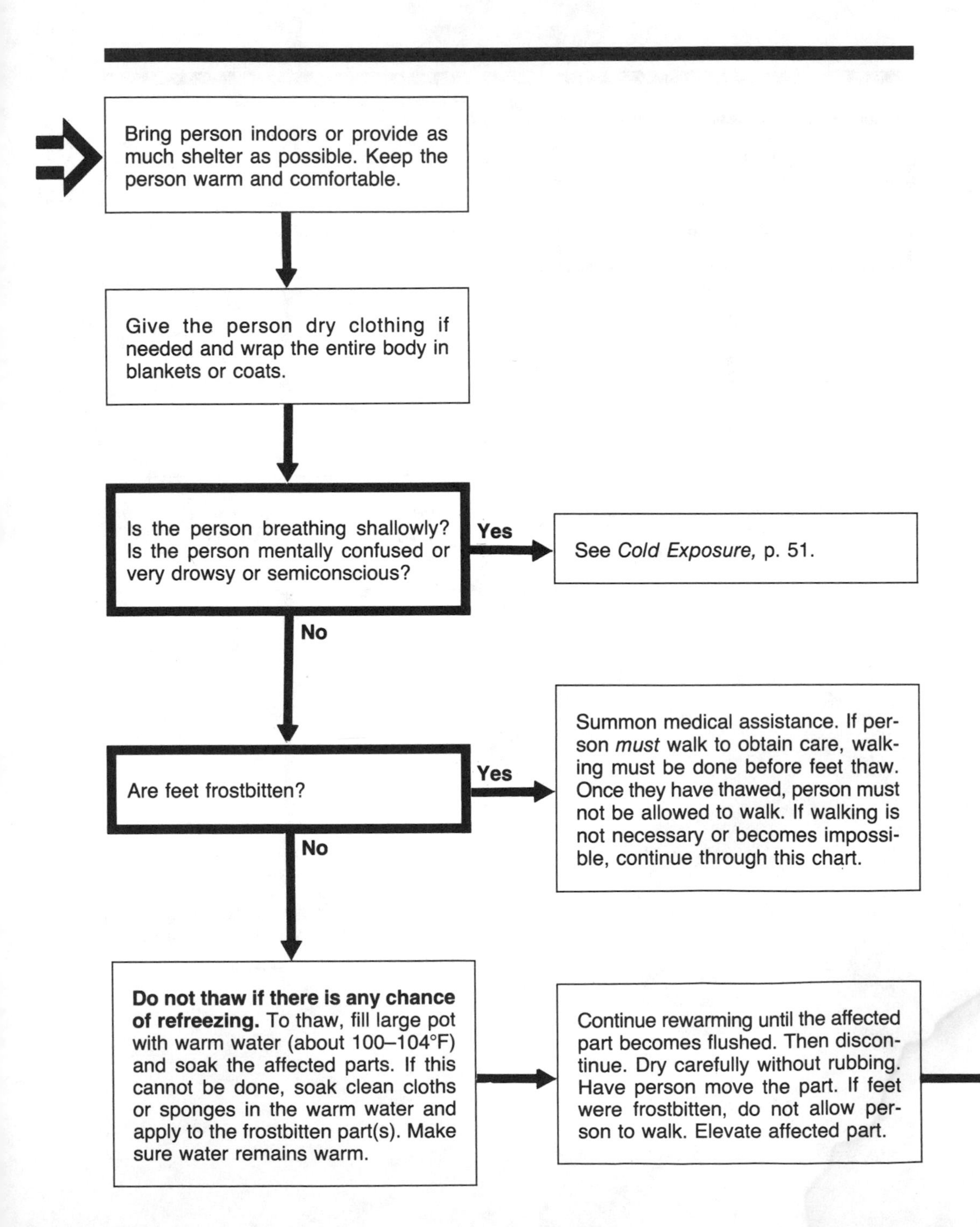
Bring person indoors or provide as much shelter as possible. Keep the person warm and comfortable.
Give the person dry clothing if needed and wrap the entire body in blankets or coats.
Is the person breathing shallowly? Is the person mentally confused or very drowsy or semiconscious?
Yes
See Cold Exposure, p. 51.
No
Are feet frostbitten?
Yes
Summon medical assistance. If person must walk to obtain care, walking must be done before feet thaw. Once they have thawed, person must not be allowed to walk. If walking is not necessary or becomes impossible, continue through this chart.
No
Do not thaw if there is any chance of refreezing. To thaw, fill large pot with warm water (about 100–104°F) and soak the affected parts. If this cannot be done, soak clean cloths or sponges in the warm water and apply to the frostbitten part(s). Make sure water remains warm.
Continue rewarming until the affected part becomes flushed. Then discontinue. Dry carefully without rubbing. Have person move the part. If feet were frostbitten, do not allow person to walk. Elevate affected part.

Calm the person by talking while attending to the problem. Explain what you are doing. Try not to show anxiety; act with confidence. Your calm behavior can help to reassure the injured person.

Give the person dry clothes and wrap in blankets. Thaw affected part in fresh warm water.

If fingers or toes were frostbitten, separate those affected with dry, sterile gauze or clean cloth. Elevate affected part(s) and protect from direct contact with bedclothes or other materials.

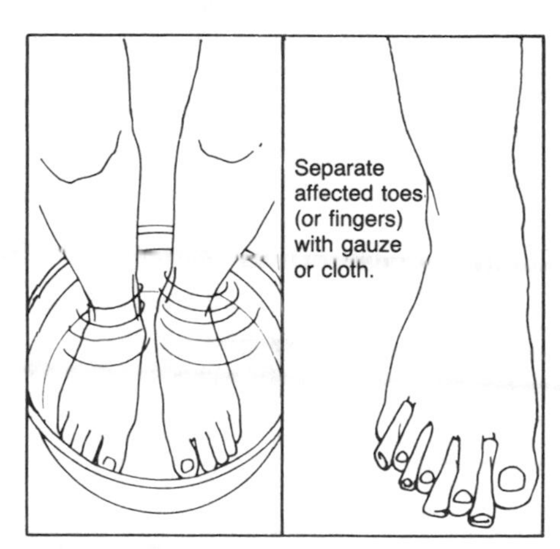
Separate affected toes (or fingers) with gauze or cloth.

Keep the person as warm and oomfortable as possible, but **not so warm that sweating occurs.**

If conscious and not vomiting, give person warm liquids to drink. **Do not give alcoholic beverages. Do not let person smoke.**

Keep the person away from sources of direct heat. If there are blisters, do not break them.

Seek medical care immediately.

53 Heat Exhaustion/ Heat Cramps

Signs & Symptoms: *cool, pale, clammy skin/fatigue and faintness/headache/ heavy sweating/weak pulse/near-normal body temperature/nausea. Onset is gradual. Person is alert.*

If person is unconscious or groggy, see *Heatstroke*, p. 54.

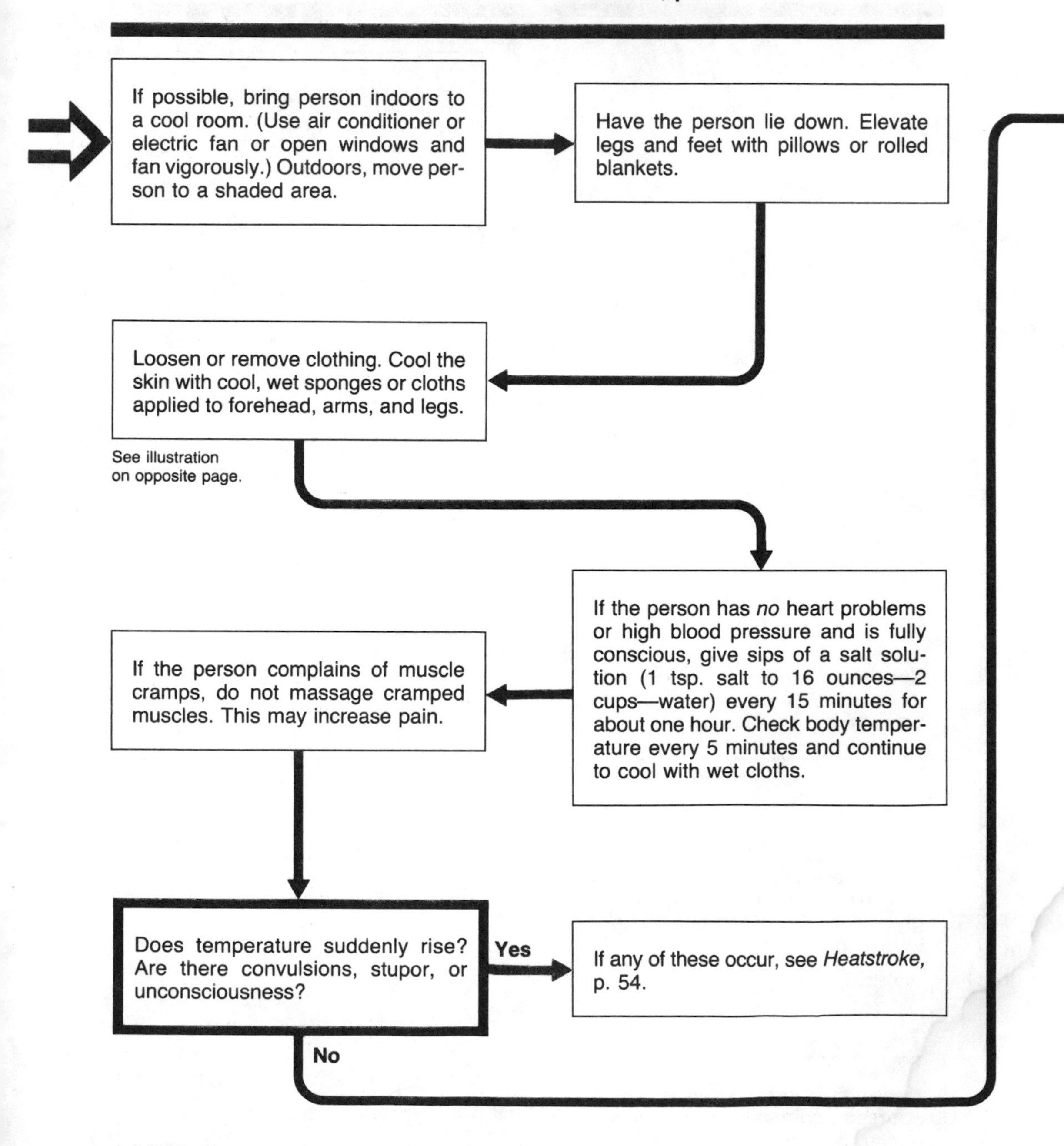

If possible, bring person indoors to a cool room. (Use air conditioner or electric fan or open windows and fan vigorously.) Outdoors, move person to a shaded area.
Have the person lie down. Elevate legs and feet with pillows or rolled blankets.
Loosen or remove clothing. Cool the skin with cool, wet sponges or cloths applied to forehead, arms, and legs.
See illustration on opposite page.
If the person has *no* heart problems or high blood pressure and is fully conscious, give sips of a salt solution (1 tsp. salt to 16 ounces—2 cups—water) every 15 minutes for about one hour. Check body temperature every 5 minutes and continue to cool with wet cloths.
If the person complains of muscle cramps, do not massage cramped muscles. This may increase pain.
Does temperature suddenly rise? Are there convulsions, stupor, or unconsciousness?
Yes
If any of these occur, see *Heatstroke*, p. 54.
No

Calm the person by talking while attending to the problem. Explain what you are doing. Try not to show anxiety; act with confidence. Your calm behavior can help to reassure the sick person.

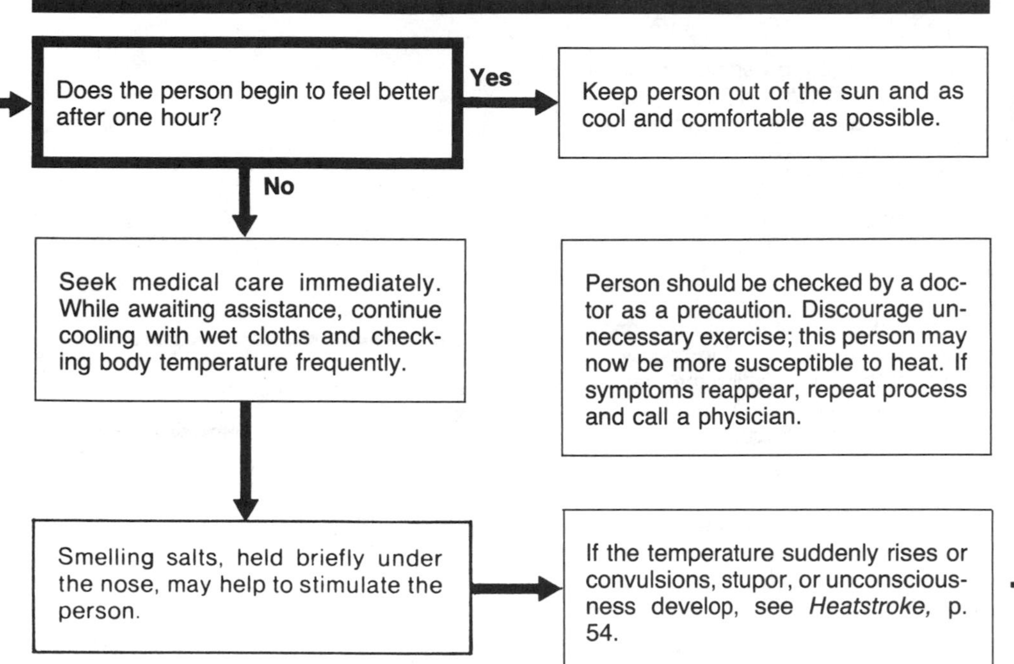
Does the person begin to feel better after one hour?
Yes
Keep person out of the sun and as cool and comfortable as possible.
No
Seek medical care immediately. While awaiting assistance, continue cooling with wet cloths and checking body temperature frequently.
Person should be checked by a doctor as a precaution. Discourage unnecessary exercise; this person may now be more susceptible to heat. If symptoms reappear, repeat process and call a physician.
Smelling salts, held briefly under the nose, may help to stimulate the person.
If the temperature suddenly rises or convulsions, stupor, or unconsciousness develop, see *Heatstroke,* p. 54.

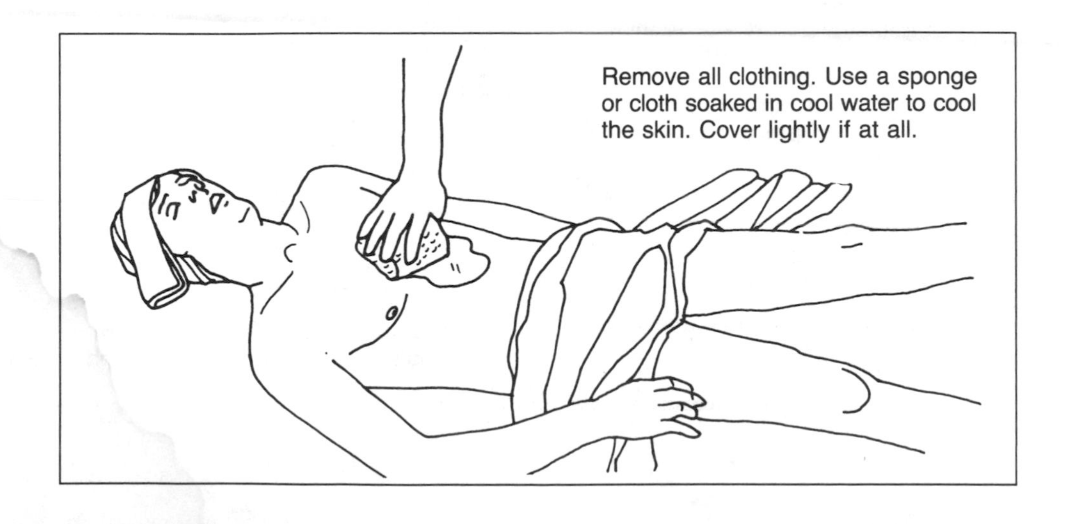
Remove all clothing. Use a sponge or cloth soaked in cool water to cool the skin. Cover lightly if at all.

Heatstroke

Signs & Symptoms: *red, hot, dry skin/no perspiration/body temperature around 106°F (very warm to the touch)/rapid pulse/stupor or unconsciousness*

If there are two or more rescuers, one should obtain emergency assistance while the other is following the procedures outlined below.

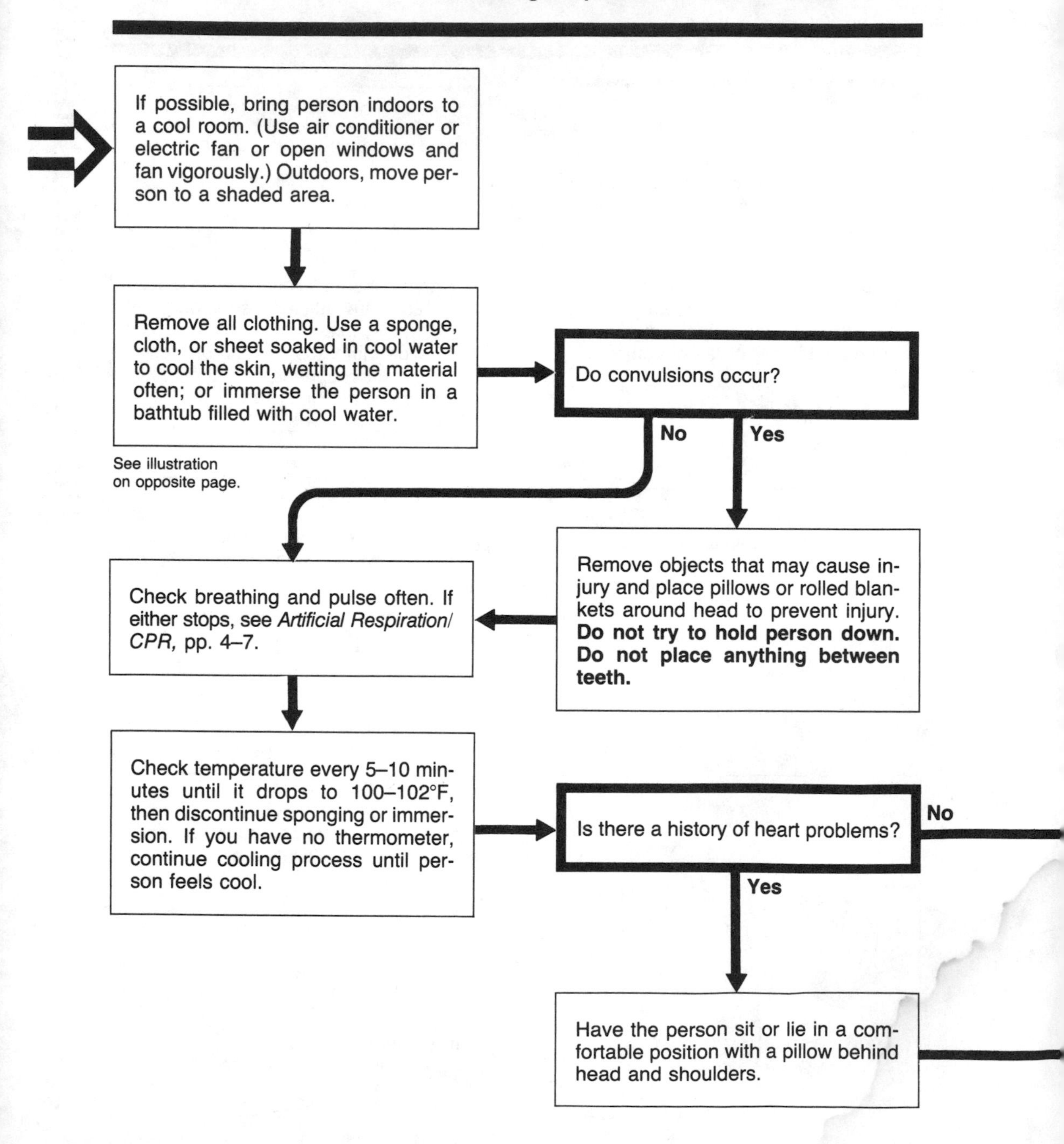

If possible, bring person indoors to a cool room. (Use air conditioner or electric fan or open windows and fan vigorously.) Outdoors, move person to a shaded area.
Remove all clothing. Use a sponge, cloth, or sheet soaked in cool water to cool the skin, wetting the material often; or immerse the person in a bathtub filled with cool water.
See illustration on opposite page.
Do convulsions occur?
No
Yes
Remove objects that may cause injury and place pillows or rolled blankets around head to prevent injury. Do not try to hold person down. Do not place anything between teeth.
Check breathing and pulse often. If either stops, see Artificial Respiration/CPR, pp. 4–7.
Check temperature every 5–10 minutes until it drops to 100–102°F, then discontinue sponging or immersion. If you have no thermometer, continue cooling process until person feels cool.
Is there a history of heart problems?
No
Yes
Have the person sit or lie in a comfortable position with a pillow behind head and shoulders.

Calm the person by talking while attending to the problem. Explain what you are doing. Try not to show anxiety; act with confidence. Your calm behavior can help to reassure the sick person.

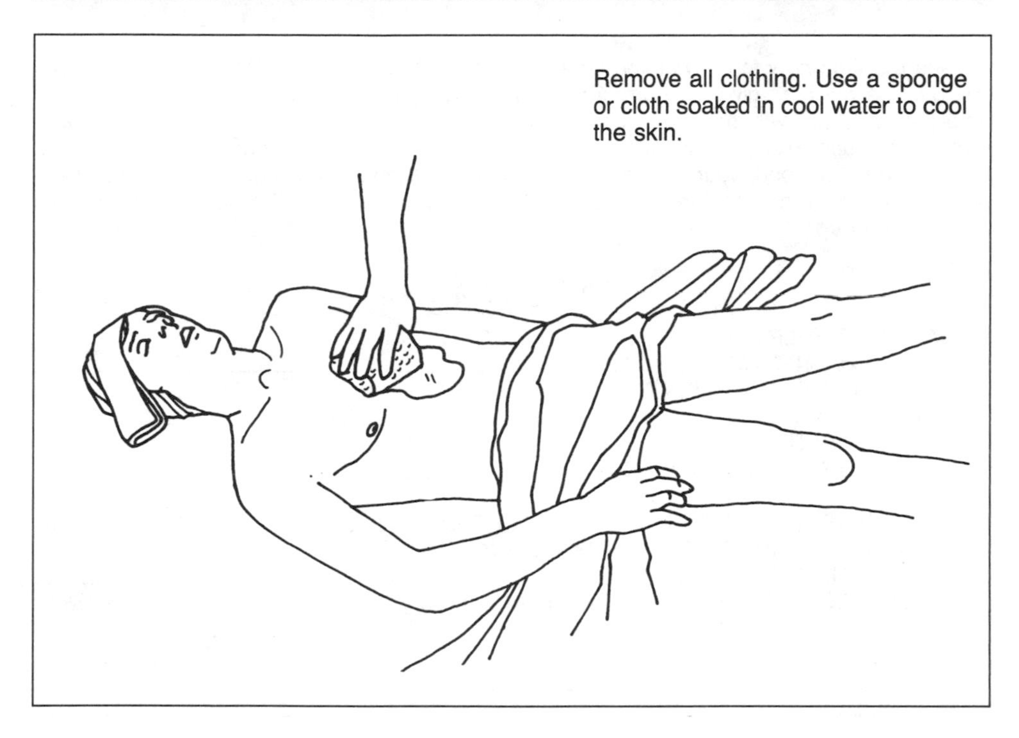

Remove all clothing. Use a sponge or cloth soaked in cool water to cool the skin.

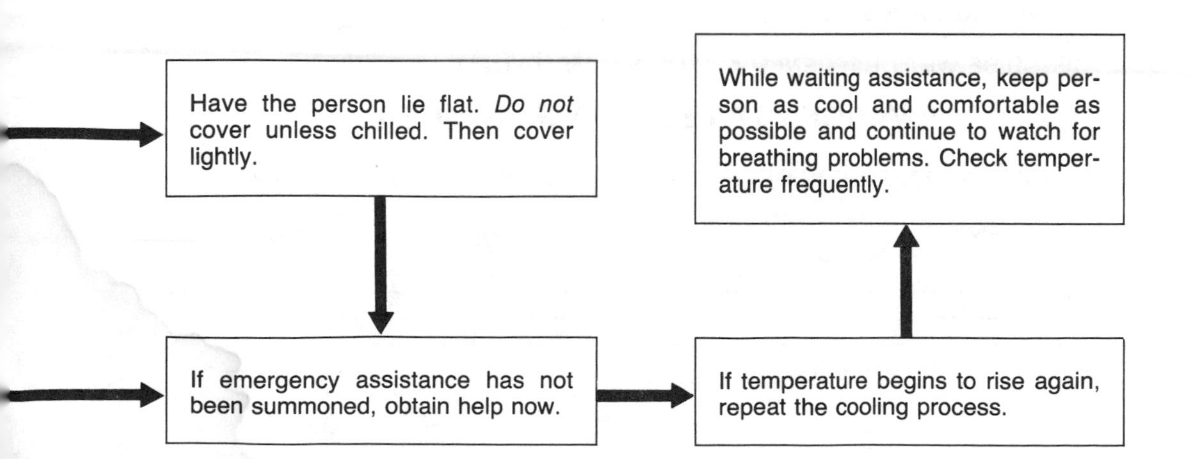
Have the person lie flat. *Do not* cover unless chilled. Then cover lightly.
If emergency assistance has not been summoned, obtain help now.
If temperature begins to rise again, repeat the cooling process.
While waiting assistance, keep person as cool and comfortable as possible and continue to watch for breathing problems. Check temperature frequently.

55 How to Get Help Fast

Take the time *now* to fill in all the necessary information on this and the following pages so you'll be ready to give the correct information as quickly and calmly as possible in an emergency. What will the dispatcher need to know? First, the location of the accident. Besides the address, you should have available directions to your home or business from a major road. Second, your phone number in case he has to call back. Third, what happened and how many people need help. Stay on the phone until the dispatcher says it's okay to hang up.

AT HOME

1. CALL FOR HELP.

P **EMERGENCY MEDICAL SERVICES** ______________________
H **FIRE DEPARTMENT** ______________________
O **POLICE** ______________________
N **HOSPITAL** ______________________
E **POISON CONTROL CENTER** ______________________

2. STATE THE ADDRESS OF THE ACCIDENT OR ILLNESS AND GIVE DIRECTIONS TO IT FROM A MAJOR ROAD—INCLUDING CROSS STREETS.
YOUR ADDRESS: ______________________
DIRECTIONS TO YOUR HOUSE OR APARTMENT—SCENE OF THE ACCIDENT:
____
____
____
____

3. WHEN ASKED, GIVE YOUR PHONE NUMBER(S) AND A NEIGHBOR'S.
YOUR PHONE NUMBER: ______________________
YOUR NEIGHBOR'S: ______________________

4. DESCRIBE WHAT HAPPENED AND HOW MANY PEOPLE NEED HELP.

EMERGENCY TELEPHONE NUMBERS

NAMES AND NUMBERS OF NEIGHBORS TRAINED IN CPR AND FIRST AID

NAME	PHONE	TRAINING

PHYSICIANS

	NAME	OFFICE PHONE	HOME PHONE
FAMILY DOCTOR			
PEDIATRICIAN			
SPECIALIST(S)			
DENTIST			

HOSPITAL EMERGENCY ROOM ______________________________

DRUGSTORE ______________________________

HUSBAND'S PHONE AT WORK ____________ WIFE'S PHONE AT WORK ____________

OTHER FAMILY MEMBER'S NUMBERS

NAME	WORK/SCHOOL	PHONE

NEIGHBORS AND FRIENDS

NAME	ADDRESS	PHONE

TAXI ______________________________

AT WORK

1. CALL FOR HELP.

EMERGENCY MEDICAL SERVICES ____________

COMPANY MEDICAL ROOM ____________

FIRE DEPARTMENT ____________

POLICE ____________

PERSONNEL DEPARTMENT ____________

COMPANY SECURITY ____________

SUPERVISOR ____________

2. STATE THE ADDRESS AND LOCATION OF THE COMPANY, INCLUDING CROSS STREETS AND SPECIFIC DIRECTIONS TO YOUR DEPARTMENT FROM THE MAIN ENTRANCE.

YOUR COMPANY'S ADDRESS: ____________

DIRECTIONS TO YOUR COMPANY: ____________

____

____

____

DIRECTIONS TO YOUR DEPARTMENT:________________________

3. GIVE YOUR PHONE NUMBER AND THE NUMBER OF A NEARBY PHONE.
   YOUR PHONE NUMBER AND EXTENSION: ____________
   PHONE NUMBER AND EXTENSION OF NEARBY PHONE (list location):________

4. DESCRIBE WHAT HAPPENED AND HOW MANY PEOPLE NEED HELP.

EMPLOYEES TRAINED IN FIRST AID AND/OR CPR

NAME	DEPARTMENT	PHONE	TRAINING

ON THE ROAD

1. CALL FOR HELP

	EMERGENCY MEDICAL SERVICES	FIRE	POLICE
HOMETOWN			
AREAS YOU VISIT REGULARLY			

EMERGENCY PHONE NUMBERS

AUTO CLUB____________
TOWING SERVICES____________
AUTO REPAIR____________
TAXI____________
AUTOMOBILE INSURANCE COMPANY____________
POLICY NUMBER____________

2. STATE THE LOCATION OF THE ACCIDENT, GIVING DIRECTIONS FROM MAJOR ROAD, INCLUDING CROSS STREETS.
3. GIVE YOUR NUMBER.
4. DESCRIBE WHAT HAPPENED AND HOW MANY PEOPLE NEED HELP. STAY ON THE LINE UNTIL DISPATCHER SAYS IT'S ALL RIGHT TO HANG UP!!!